PRAISE FOR LAUGHTER YOGA

'Laughter yoga is a perfect way to laugh and get exercise at the same time. It approaches laughter as a body exercise, so it's easy to laugh even if you're depressed or in a bad mood . . . I've tried it, and it works.'
Oprah Winfrey

'I can't think of any other body – mind technique that has caught on this way. I told [the] American Senate Committee during a hearing about health-care reform that laughter yoga could help lower American health-care costs.'
Dr Andrew Weil

'Laughter yoga exemplifies a form of "right-brain thinking" that managers should promote.'
Daniel H. Pink, *New York Times* **bestselling author of** *A Whole New Mind*

'Laughter connects you with people. It's almost impossible to maintain any kind of distance or any sense of social hierarchy when you're just howling with laughter. Laughter is a force for democracy.'
John Cleese, after visiting a laughter club in Mumbai during the filming of the BBC's TV series *The Human Face*

LAUGHTER YOGA

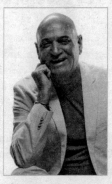

Dr Madan Kataria, popularly known as 'the guru of giggling' (*The Times*), is the founder of the laughter yoga club movement that started in 1995 in Mumbai. A sought-after keynote and motivational speaker for corporations and organizations around the world, he has conducted seminars and workshops for UBS, Emirates Bank, IBM, Hewlett-Packard, and Volvo, among many others. He has also been featured on *The Oprah Winfrey Show*, CNN, and ABC, and is associated with an increasing number of medical research projects analyzing the benefits of laughter. Retired from medical practice, he devotes all his time to writing, teaching, coaching, and training laughter leaders in order to foster the spread of laughter clubs. He is the creator of the immensely popular World Laughter Day, which is celebrated on the first Sunday of every May.

Dr Andrew Weil is the *New York Times* bestselling author of numerous books, including *Spontaneous Happiness*, *Spontaneous Healing*, and *Healthy Aging*. A world-renowned pioneer in the field of integrative medicine, he is the founder and director of the Arizona Center for Integrative Medicine at the University of Arizona Health Sciences Center.

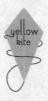

LAUGHTER YOGA

Daily Practices FOR Health AND Happiness

Dr MADAN KATARIA

FOREWORD BY Dr Andrew Weil

yellow kite

First published in Great Britain in 2020 by Yellow Kite
An Imprint of Hodder & Stoughton
An Hachette UK company

First published in India in 2018 by Ebury Press
Part of Penguin Random House India

First published in the United States in 2020
Published by arrangement with Penguin
An imprint of Penguin Random House LLC

This paperback edition published in 2021

1

Paperback ISBN 978 1 529 31110 5
eBook ISBN 978 1 529 30806 8

Printed and bound in Great Britain by Clays Ltd, Elcograf S.p.A.

Hodder & Stoughton policy is to use papers that are natural, renewable and recyclable products and made from wood grown in sustainable forests. The logging and manufacturing processes are expected to conform to the environmental regulations of the country of origin.

Yellow Kite
Hodder & Stoughton Ltd
Carmelite House
50 Victoria Embankment
London EC4Y 0DZ

www.yellowkitebooks.co.uk

To all my students,
from whom I learned more than what I taught

When you laugh, you change,
and when you change, the world changes.

Contents

Foreword

The success of laughter yoga and scientific studies across the world have left no doubt that laughter has a powerful and profound effect on the human body and mind. Not only does it help to prevent illnesses but also contributes toward healing chronic diseases—both physical and mental. Unfortunately, most people are unaware of the benefits of laughter if practiced regularly. Until Dr Madan Kataria made laughter yoga popular both in India and globally, there was no reliable method of bringing more laughter into people's lives. His breakthrough has allowed people to enjoy the many benefits of laughter without depending on external conditions and stimulation. It employs a remarkable exercise routine that combines yogic breathing with laughter, making it an ideal tool for complete body-mind wellness.

The method is straightforward. After brief physical and breathing exercises under the direction of a trained individual, people simulate laughter with vigorous repetitions of 'ha ha' and 'ho ho.' This fake laughter soon becomes real and contagious and may even continue for half an hour or more.

Laughter increases the supply of oxygen to body tissues, boosts immunity, relieves pain, lowers stress and even helps protect against heart disease, diabetes, arthritis, migraine and cancer. It is a powerful technique: safe, easy and a lot of fun.

I can't think of any other body-mind technique that has caught on in this way. As laughter yoga gains popularity worldwide, the experience of thousands of people has stimulated research on the physiology and neurochemistry of laughter. I believe the movement is contributing significantly to public health.

Mere knowledge about laughter is not enough; you must practice it. It is the regular practice of unconditional laughter that brings about the desired physiological and biochemical changes that sustain a positive mental attitude. Training yourself to laugh regularly can also increase genuineness, compassion and sensitivity. It can make you more effective in dealing with others and with everyday situations. Over time, laughter yoga engenders qualities that can help you live a more sensible and virtuous life.

Dr Andrew Weil
Tucson, Arizona

Introduction

This book is a testament to my journey with laughter yoga, which began in India in 1995 with only five people and has reached over 100 countries today. Not only has laughter changed my life dramatically, it has also touched the lives of many others around the world.

The way laughter yoga has been growing exponentially without any marketing or advertisement indicates how effective and powerful it is. Laughter yoga is not rocket science—it is simple but profound. In fact, this unique concept has redefined laughter. Most people knew that laughter was the best medicine for the body and mind, but there was never a reliable delivery system. Laughter was simply the end result of some entertainment or amusement. Laughter yoga took it to an all-new level with a complete delivery system that allowed laughter to be prescribed as part of a daily routine in order to realize all the health benefits it has to offer.

The concept of laughing for no reason stems from my roots. The youngest of eight children, I grew up in a small farming village, Mohrewala, in Punjab. It was here that I learned about the relationship between simplicity and laughter. Most people in the village could laugh at the smallest of things. They did not need a reason to laugh or share jokes. For them, laughter was the most natural outcome of their uncomplicated daily lives. Meeting each other and dancing and singing at festivals, weddings and celebrations was reason enough to laugh and have fun. However, my perception of people and their ability to laugh underwent a major change while studying medicine in a big city.

Life was different in a metropolis. People were alone, constantly battling the stresses of modern life. Not having many reasons to laugh, they were always on the lookout for one. Their happiness and laughter were primarily conditional. Laughter was no longer natural; it was dependent on logic and reason. Also, people were self-conscious about laughing. Often, their laughter and humor turned negative as they ridiculed others.

Soon, I began my pursuit of laughter and happiness. The search for unconditional laughter led me to the discovery of laughter yoga, which guarantees benefits for everyone, even those who are serious and introverted. Never in my wildest dreams had I imagined that laughter could be as simple as that: just laugh, because you can!

This book begins with the history and genesis of the laughter yoga phenomenon: how it evolved and spread across the globe, spilling into different areas of life. You will learn how to practice laughter exercises in groups, as couples, and even by yourself. Laughing for no reason is the concept and philosophy behind the methods of laughter yoga. This idea can be used to put to rest many myths and misconceptions about laughter. For example, it answers questions such as: How can you laugh when you don't feel like it? How can you laugh if you are not happy? Do you need a sense of humor to laugh? Why do children laugh so much and adults so little? How can I learn to laugh?

The benefits of laughter are numerous in all facets of life— personal, professional and social. Backed by countless evidence-based studies, laughter is practiced not only as an exercise but also as a therapeutic tool to control chronic diseases.

Many regular practitioners of laughter yoga have shared their life-changing experiences in this book. This book also includes several scientific studies, based on laughter methods, that have been conducted in universities all over the world.

Laughter yoga was conceived when the world needed it, at a time when everyday life was becoming more stressful and stress-relieving methods were becoming time-consuming, complicated or expensive. Over the years, yogic laughter has helped me uncover the principles of the inner spirit of laughter. My personal stories, based on my belief system of sensible and virtuous living, will hopefully motivate and inspire the reader to cultivate a more positive mental attitude, which will enable him/her to get past the challenges of life with a smile.

Finally, the practical suggestions about strategies and tools in this book will assist the reader in bringing more laughter into his/her daily life.

Laughter yoga is instant yoga. Its benefits can be felt from the very first session. Not just this, it is cost-effective, less time-consuming, has scientific backing and is easy to learn.

Keep laughing! Ha ha!

Find Your Laughter Quotient

How much do you laugh each day? Do you laugh enough? Is laughter all about laughing? Not at all. Complete this questionnaire and find your Laughter Quotient (LQ). Once you calculate your LQ, you can decide how to bring more laughter and joy into your life and into the lives of those around you.

Rate each question/statement on a scale of 1–5:

> 1: Not true at all
> 2: Slightly true
> 3: Moderately true
> 4: Mostly true
> 5: Absolutely true

1. I laugh a lot every day.
   1   2   3   4   5

2. My laughter is driven by my internal desire to laugh and have fun.
   1   2   3   4   5

3. I use humor each day to perceive, express and experience situations in a humorous way.
   1   2   3   4   5

4. I am very playful, both physically and mentally, while interacting with others.
   1   2   3   4   5

5. I sing for no reason.
   1   2   3   4   5

6. I dance for no reason.
   1   2   3   4   5

7. I freely express positive and negative emotions.
   1   2   3   4   5

8. I have a high percentage of positive thoughts.
   1   2   3   4   5

9. I am peaceful and calm most of the time.
   1   2   3   4   5

10. I frequently feel excited and passionate about life.
    1   2   3   4   5

11. I often express myself as an extrovert.
    1   2   3   4   5

12. I am satisfied and happy with life.
    1   2   3   4   5

13. My physical, mental and emotional state is mostly relaxed.
    1   2   3   4   5

14. I am able to communicate and interact with strangers with ease.
    1   2   3   4   5

15. I generally feel refreshed and energetic.
    1   2   3   4   5

16. I stay positive during challenging times.
    1   2   3   4   5

17. I stay connected with friends.
    1   2   3   4   5

18. It is easy for me to laugh without a reason.
    1   2   3   4   5

19. I often perform random acts of kindness.
    1   2   3   4   5

20. I have the ability to act silly before others.
    1   2   3   4   5

If your score is:

80–100: You laugh a lot. Keep it up!
60–79: You are good at laughing, but you can do better.
40–59: You laugh very little and need to be happier.
Under 40: You seem to have a serious problem and must do something to bring more laughter into your life.

Part I

ORIGIN

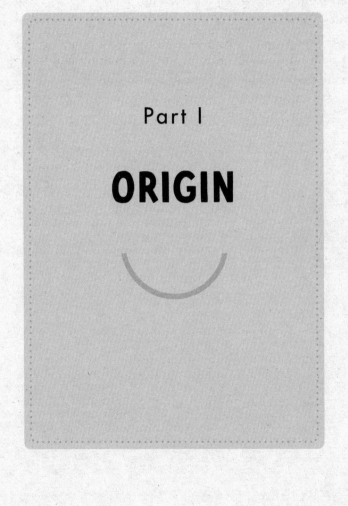

1

Origins of Laughter Yoga

*"The sun demands no reason to shine, water demands
no reason to flow, a child demands no reason to smile,
then why do we need a reason to laugh?"*

My Laughter Story

Born in a small village on the India-Pakistan border, I was the youngest of eight children. Hailing from a farming background, my parents had never attended school. Being simple village folk, they were mostly engrossed in the daily grind of farm life. None of my siblings were interested in academics, which made me the odd one out. It was my mother's dream that I become a doctor because in those days one had to travel almost ten miles to seek any kind of medical help. She hoped that I would study medicine and return to the village.

In pursuance of her wish, I went to a boarding school in Ferozepur, Punjab, and got my medical degree from Amritsar Medical College. After graduating, I went to Mumbai and started practicing as a family physician. Lured by the glitz and glitterati of the city, I imagined myself becoming rich and famous. I tried everything I could to reach for the skies, but soon realized that it was not that simple. I did not succeed in my quest and slumped into depression.

Life was tough as it was not easy to make money without any experience. I was stressed and miserable. My mother, who visited Mumbai at that point, was shocked to see my state. "Madan, what is wrong? You don't look happy and you don't laugh and smile like you used to in the village," she would ask.

She was right. Somewhere in the midst of the hurried upward scramble to the imagined riches, I had lost my laughter. The transition from an innocent village boy to a city doctor had altered my persona. Having realized the enormity of the situation, I embarked on a new search, and this time it was not money. It was to find my laughter again: the key to happiness and joy.

Not content with being just a physician in a suburb of Mumbai, I launched a health magazine called *My Doctor* to spread more awareness about the importance of good health. It was in March 1995, while writing an article titled "Laughter: The Best Medicine" for my magazine, that I stumbled upon a rich repertoire of scientific work done on laughter as a therapy. Further exploration led me to an amazing volume of documented studies that described many proven benefits of laughter on the mind and body.

While going through all the scientific literature, I was profoundly inspired by *Anatomy of an Illness*, a book by American journalist Norman Cousins. It describes how Cousins laughed his way back to health from ankylosing spondylitis, a chronic condition affecting the spine. He took a lot of painkillers each day but found no relief, which is why he decided to watch funny movies instead. To his surprise, he found that just thirty minutes of laughter gave him almost two hours of painless sleep.

I also read about the scientific studies conducted by Dr. Lee Berk of Loma Linda University in California, which showed that mirthful laughter reduced stress and had a positive impact on the immune system.

This got me thinking. Life in Mumbai was stressful and people hardly laughed. They were forever in a rush and struggled to meet their needs and fulfill their dreams. Even I appeared dour and had lost my laughter to the daily rigors of my profession and the added burden of a publication. It was not a joke: there was no time to laugh.

I believed that laughter could improve health and enable one to cope with the stressors of the modern age. I looked for ways to add more laughter to people's lives and help them with their medical or personal crises. I started joking and laughing with my patients and realized that they recovered much faster when they were happy and positive.

The Beginning

It was March 13, 1995. I was awake at 4 a.m. and pacing up and down my living room, desperate to find a solution to the stress I was facing. An idea came to me: if laughter was indeed so good, why not set up a laughter club? I was ecstatic and could hardly wait to implement the concept. Three hours later, I hurried to the public park where I went for a morning walk every day. I tried to convince a few regular walkers about the importance of laughter and the idea of starting a laughter club.

The response was predictable. They were nonplussed and probably thought that I was crazy. They laughed at the idea and scoffed at the concept. But I persisted and managed to motivate 4 out of 400 people. The first laughter club started with just five people.

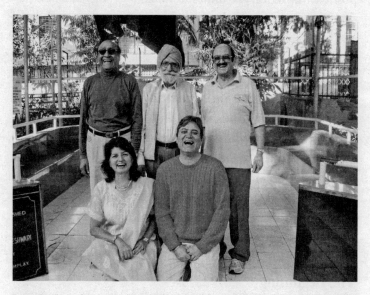

L to R: (standing) Madan Mohan Pushkarna, Mohan Singh, Rajendra Tandon; (sitting) Madhuri and Dr. Madan Kataria. They were members of the first laughter club in 1995.

We met for half an hour every morning to laugh together, much to the amusement of befuddled onlookers. Initially, the sessions would begin with someone sharing a joke or a humorous anecdote. Soon, we started enjoying the whole exercise and reported feeling much better after a laughter session of just twenty to thirty minutes.

Despite the initial ridicule and criticism, I continued to advocate the health benefits laughter had to offer. Gradually, more people became receptive and showed interest. The numbers rose and by the end of the week there were nearly fifty-five people. The routine continued with much vigor for the next ten days, after which we hit a snag. The good jokes and stories were replaced by negative and hurtful ones. Reacting to the offensive jokes, two members complained that it would be better to close the club. Determined to keep the laughter club alive, I asked the members to give me a day to resolve the crisis. That night, I looked up methods to laugh without jokes. Luckily, I chanced upon a book called *Emotions and Health* from the Prevention Health Care Series. As I read a chapter on humor and laughter, I was surprised to learn that the body cannot differentiate between real and fake laughter. It concluded that if one could not manage a genuine laugh, one should pretend to do so. I also learned that not only laughter but a bodily expression of any motion generates a similar emotion in the mind. This was the breakthrough I was looking for: why not use laughter as an exercise?

The next morning, I explained the concept to the group and asked them to act like they were laughing for a minute. Though skeptical, they agreed. The results were amazing. For some, the fake laughter quickly turned into real laughter. It was contagious. Soon, the others followed. The group laughed like never before with hearty laughter continuing for almost ten minutes.

Finally, there was laughter, real laughter with no jokes.

The fact that one could laugh without an external trigger was something unique. However, there were some people who were shy and found it difficult to laugh without a reason. As every person has a different psychological makeup, it is harder for some people to laugh at will. My new challenge was to get these people to laugh.

I came up with warm-up exercises like clapping and chanting "ho ho" and "ha ha ha." This helped people laugh more easily. Soon, varied laughter exercises were developed, which included elements of role play like childlike playfulness and other techniques from my theater days.

As the concept evolved, I identified similarities between laughter and pranayama. Both of them are based on the principle of optimal breathing, which is fundamental to good health. Together with my wife, Madhuri, I incorporated elements from this ancient form of yogic breathing into laughter. The result was laughter yoga or *hasya* yoga—a complete workout for health and wellness. A physically oriented technique, it offers multiple health benefits, primarily increasing the supply of oxygen to all parts of the body and boosting the immune system. It also energizes metabolism.

Scores of people are now taking advantage of the numerous benefits of laughter and experiencing relief from a variety of stress-related illnesses. Today, laughter has grown on its own strength. It is undoubtedly nature's best medicine.

Initial Challenges

As I look back, I recall how the laughter club started for fun. I had never dreamed that it would become such a big movement. In its initial days, it was quite difficult for me to get started. The fear of being laughed at made people apprehensive of joining the group. In fact, the first one to object was the caretaker of the garden where we started the first laughter club. It was thought of as a public nuisance and I was advised to discontinue. However, I continued to motivate people. It was after a few talks on the health benefits of laughter that people started coming forward. Even then, many ridiculed the idea and called us *murakh mandli*, which means "a band of fools" in Hindi. Of the 300 to 400 people who came to walk in the Lokhandwala Park in Mumbai's Andheri (west) every day, only fifteen to twenty people joined initially. More people trickled in after they reported feeling a sense of well-being after the sessions. This made the park authorities soften their stand and allow the laughter group to continue. Soon, the number of members swelled to fifty-five and then sixty, including women.

The very idea of laughing in a public place without a reason intrigued many people, who saw an ordinary bunch of people engaged in what they perceived was a "funny" activity. People would look at us from the balconies of their houses and from the roadside. The hundreds who walked in the park couldn't resist staring as they passed us. The initial reaction was that of amusement and surprise. The question on everyone's mind was: how could we laugh in a public place without a reason? Some of those living around the spacious park half-heartedly objected to being woken up by the laughter.

Those who practiced it daily and found it beneficial began spreading the news by word of mouth. The concept rapidly caught on in the residential area and many people would come to watch the "funny" people in action. As we kept updating our laughing techniques, people from adjoining localities also expressed the desire to start similar clubs in their areas. We were only too happy to share the joy. In less than two months, sixteen laughter clubs had come up all over Mumbai.

> **Lotte Mikkelsen, London:** *I started my daily laughter practice in 2008 after I was diagnosed with multiple sclerosis (MS) and have not stopped laughing since. This has had a major impact on my health with no relapses related to MS. In addition, I find that the way I deal with life in general and with other people has become more compassionate and kind. Laughter yoga has taught me and allowed me to express tears, playfulness and unconditional laughter without judging others and myself.*

Unstoppable Laughter

Within a month, thirteen laughter clubs had come up in Mumbai. Back in my hometown, the local newspaper carried a photograph of one of the laughter clubs on the front page, which sent my eldest brother into a state of panic. He called me.

"Madan, what are you doing? Please stop it immediately. This is causing us a lot of embarrassment. We sent you to become a doctor; instead you've become a laughingstock."

I tried to explain that the club was not funny entertainment or cheap comedy—it was a health club dedicated to maintaining the well-being of its members. But all explanations were in vain. He was adamant that I stop my laughter movement.

In order to convince my family, I invited my mother and brother to Mumbai and took them to the Jogger's Park laughter club. They were surprised to see over 100 people laughing together. Most of them were professionals like doctors, engineers, accountants and businessmen. Coming from a small town where women were usually too shy to participate in any public activity, they were amazed to see even women actively take part in the sessions.

The overwhelming response from the members and the feeling of harmony displayed at the sessions had a profound impact on my family and they changed their attitude about the laughter movement. Comprehending the tremendous health benefits and the happiness and joy that the clubs have instilled in people across the world, they now take pride in my work and are part of my laughter family.

2

What Is Laughter Yoga and
Why Do We Need It?

"We have taken life too seriously.
Now, it's time to take laughter seriously."

Why Do We Need to Laugh More Today?

Over the past four decades, scientific research has proved that laughter has a profound effect on our bodies and minds. People have forgotten to laugh and consequently they frequently fall sick. Maintaining good health has become a challenge, but laughter yoga has come to the rescue of thousands in coping with stress and dealing with difficulties with a smile.

Stress: The No. 1 Killer

Laughter is fast disappearing from our high-pressure, high-tension modern world. Most illnesses today, be it high blood pressure, heart diseases, anxiety, depression, frequent coughs and colds, nervous breakdowns, peptic ulcers, insomnia, allergies, asthma, irritable bowel syndrome, colitis, menstrual abnormalities, migraine and even cancer, are stress-related. People find it difficult to laugh amidst these endless stressors. Though there are many methods available to release stress, most of them are time-consuming and expensive. Laughter yoga is cost-effective and the fastest way to reduce stress. The technique itself is simple and everyone can practice it.

Depression: The No. 1 Sickness

According to the World Health Organization (WHO), 300 million people suffer from depression worldwide. It is the leading cause of disability and affects over 15 million American adults, or about 6.7 percent of the U.S. population that is above the age of eighteen in a given year.[1]

Trying to cope with life's challenges, people often find themselves alone. With no one to talk to or share their feelings with, they sink into depression. This despondency is growing rapidly and has become the no. 1 sickness in the world. If you observe closely, you will find many elderly people in old-age homes who are depressed and youngsters who find it hard to deal with their careers or relationships. The number of suicides is on the rise and the inability to express emotions is becoming a cause for concern.

Laughter is a powerful antidote to depression as it releases endorphins, or the feel-good hormone, and increases the levels of dopamine and serotonin, which help maintain a good mood. Depressed people laugh rarely, but with laughter yoga one is less likely to be depressed.

Helga, Norway: *I have been laughing daily for some years now which has helped me master my life in a much better way. I laugh alone every morning while driving to work. It takes about ten to fifteen minutes, and by the time I reach my office I'm in a fantastic mood. Nothing brings me down, which proves to be very helpful as I work with people who are sick. Every day, I write the words "ha ha" on my left hand, which serve as an important reminder for me to laugh when it's not the obvious thing to do. For instance, if I'm stressed or angry with my husband, a few laughs bring the stress down or help the anger subside. It even helps me communicate with people around. In fact, one of these days I might just get a "ha ha" tattoo done . . . Ha ha!*

An Overdose of Seriousness

Newspapers and television continuously bombard us with bad news, making us feel less secure. There is a lack of laughter even at the workplace, where it is believed that seriousness is the key to being more effective. However, this is not always true. People who are serious are usually less productive, and those who take themselves lightly are likely to be more efficient. We already pay a heavy price for taking life too seriously. It is now time to take laughter seriously. Laughter yoga can prove to be the tool that helps people loosen up and prepares them to take on all challenges.

Expensive Modern Medicine

Life expectancy has increased significantly thanks to advanced medical, surgical and diagnostic techniques. But for most people in developing countries, medical treatment remains expensive and beyond reach.

Laughter is preventive and has therapeutic value. It can help cut down on medical expenses by strengthening the immune system and reducing the risk of stress-related diseases.

People Have Forgotten How to Laugh

Where is our laughter? Who do you see laughing? Doesn't it seem like people have forgotten how to laugh.

Children can laugh up to 400 times in a day, but for adults this frequency drops to barely 15 times a day. Children laugh more than adults because they do not place conditions on laughter. They laugh because they want to and because they are intrinsically joyful. As we grow older, we set conditions that limit our laughter. For example, if I get this, I will laugh, or if I get a job I like, I will be happy. We always look for reasons to laugh, but unfortunately there are few situations that make us laugh genuinely. In fact, there are an increasing number of circumstances that leave us unhappy.

Most people rely on four things to laugh: level of happiness, satisfaction, sense of humor and reason. However, these factors are unreliable as it is unlikely that we will always be happy. The million-dollar question is: how can we find laughter despite all odds, and who will make us laugh?

Laughter Yoga: A Unique Exercise Routine

Laughter yoga combines unconditional laughter with yogic breathing—pranayama. It helps people laugh without relying

on humor, jokes or comedy. Laughter is initially simulated
as a physical exercise while maintaining eye contact with the
others in the group and promoting childlike playfulness. In
most cases, this leads to real laughter. Science has proved
that the body cannot differentiate between simulated and
real laughter. Laughter yoga is the only technique that allows
adults to laugh heartily without involving cognitive thought.
It bypasses the intellectual system that normally acts as a
brake on natural laughter.

Laughter yoga sessions start with gentle warm-up
movements that include stretching, chanting and clapping.
These reduce inhibitions and help cultivate childlike
playfulness.

Breathing exercises are used to prepare the lungs,
followed by a series of laughter exercises that combine the
acting and visualization techniques with playfulness. These
exercises, when combined with the strong social dynamics
of group behavior, lead to hearty unconditional laughter.
The laughter exercises themselves are interspersed with
breathing exercises. It has been scientifically proved that just
twenty minutes of laughter each day is sufficient to enjoy the
physiological benefits it offers.

A laughter yoga session may finish with laughter
meditation, during which participants sit or lie down and
allow natural laughter to flow. This is a powerful experience
of unstructured laughter that often leads to healthy emotional
catharsis and a feeling of joy that can last for days. This can be
followed by guided relaxation exercises.

Since laughter yoga approaches laughter as an exercise,
it can be prescribed and practiced by everyone irrespective

of cultural background, language and state of mind. In fact, laughter yoga is fast catching on and is now practiced in companies, old-age homes, schools, colleges, fitness centers, community centers, prisons, hospitals, homes for the physically and mentally challenged and cancer self-help groups.

Three Reasons to Practice Laughter Yoga

Many people ask why they should force themselves to laugh when jokes or comedy films can do the trick.

Here are three reasons why one must try laughter yoga:

- **Laughter Should Be Sustained:** In order to enjoy the health benefits of laughter, one needs to laugh for at least ten to fifteen minutes each day. In other words, it should be sustained laughter. As natural laughter barely lasts for more than three to four seconds at a time, it is not sufficient to bring about physiological and psychological changes in our bodies. Since laughter becomes an exercise in laughter yoga, one can prolong it for as long as one wants. This brings with it measurable physiological changes like increased oxygen levels in the blood, relaxed muscles, better blood circulation and the release of certain hormones.

- **Laughter Should Be Deep:** To reap the health benefits of laughter, it has to be hearty and deep, coming from the diaphragm. It should be a belly laugh. Since it might not be socially acceptable to laugh loudly in public spaces, laughter yoga clubs provide a safe environment where one can laugh loudly without any worries.

- **Laughter Should Be Unconditional:** Natural laughter
  depends on many factors, but the fact is that there are not
  many things that can make us laugh. This means that
  we invariably leave laughter to chance; it may or may not
  happen. In contrast, laughter yoga allows the participants
  to laugh unconditionally. We do not leave laughter to
  chance but do it out of commitment to enjoy its health
  benefits.

3

The Essential Link Between
Yoga and Laughter

"Laughter is the shortest distance between two people."

—Victor Borge

What does a simple emotion like laughter and a universally acclaimed form of exercise like yoga have in common? Yoga has always been distinguished as a classic system of ancient Indian philosophy because it allows greater control over the body and mind.

The word "yoga" comes from the Sanskrit root *yuj*, which means to get hold of, integrate and harmonize. It means getting a hold on our lives, integrating all aspects and harmonizing our bodies with our minds, spirits and society. Though I never thought of yoga when I conceptualized laughter clubs, as the concept evolved I identified a deep connection between the basics of yoga and what we did at the laughter clubs.

After I had managed to convince people to do ten to fifteen minutes of laughter yoga exercises each day, and to take them seriously, I realized that there were many who found it difficult to laugh. In my search for a method that would let people laugh without a reason, I introduced a warm-up exercise that involved chanting "ho ho" and "ha ha ha" in unison and focusing on the abdominal muscles. This helped shed inhibitions and ensured full participation.

One morning, as I was practicing my yogic breathing, I realized that "ho ho" and "ha ha ha" were similar to *kapalbhati*—a dynamic breathing exercise in yoga. Both laughter and kapalbhati involve rhythmic movements of the diaphragm and abdominal muscles. It then occurred to me that I should combine yogic deep breathing (pranayama) with laughter exercises. I had found a perfect blend, which I named laughter yoga or hasya yoga.

While studying yoga in depth, I discovered that breathing was a fundamental part of it. Many scientific studies have proved that deep breathing has a calming effect on the mind. This prompted me to intersperse laughter exercises with deep breathing as people can get tired of laughing continuously. This worked wonders as the participants found it to be relaxing, and it made laughter yoga seem like a fun exercise. More and more people were drawn to it as they gradually comprehended the benefits of doing yoga combined with laughter. In our busy lives, there is not much time for yogic breathing daily, but it is easy to make laughter yoga a ritual as it is effortless and fun.

Breath Is Life

Breathing is a precondition for life. One can live without food and water for days but cannot survive if breathing stops even for a few minutes. According to yogic philosophy, we are alive because the cosmic energy from the universe, which is considered to be a life-giving force, flows into our bodies when we breathe.

From a medical point of view, the most important component of breathing is oxygen. Dr. Otto Warburg, president of the Institute of Cell Physiology, Germany, and a Nobel laureate, said, "Deep-breathing techniques increase oxygen to the cells and are the most important factors in living a disease-free and energetic life. When cells get enough oxygen, cancer will not and cannot occur."[1]

Stress and a negative mental state can cause breathing to become shallow and irregular. We tend to hold our breath whenever we are upset or in a state of turmoil. This leads to accumulation of carbon dioxide in the blood that causes anxiety, stress and emotional reactions.

More Oxygen from Exhalation

The hallmark of yogic breathing is that we exhale for longer than what we inhale so as to get rid of as much residual air as possible and bring in fresh air and more oxygen for the next breathing cycle. Have you realized what we do while laughing? When we laugh, we exhale for much longer than in regular breathing. While breathing normally, we inhale and exhale only 500 milliliters of oxygen even though there are 1200 to 1500 milliliters of residual air with more carbon dioxide inside our lungs.

This stale air can be forcefully exhaled through laughter exercises that allow more oxygen to enter our bodies.

Breathing Capacity and Laughter

The principal organs of respiration are the lungs. Due to our sedentary lifestyle we do not fully utilize their capacity. As a result, a part of our lung cells does not participate in the exchange of oxygen and carbon dioxide. Laughter and deep-breathing exercises open up all the cells and the respiratory passages. This leads to an increase in breathing capacity, which is also called vital capacity.

Diaphragm Activates the Parasympathetic System

The diaphragm is a major muscle that separates the thoracic and abdominal cavities. Two-thirds of the breathing procedure happens because of the movement of the diaphragm while only one-third takes place because of the expansion of the ribcage. When stressed out, most people breathe from the chest and do not use their diaphragms.

Both laughter and yogic breathing exercises are intended to stimulate the movement of the diaphragm and the abdominal muscles. The diaphragm is connected to a special branch of the autonomic nervous system called the parasympathetic system, or the calming branch, which is responsible for relaxation. The opposite is the sympathetic system, also known as the stress arousal system. One can turn this system off simply by learning how to move the diaphragm. The most important exercise in laughter yoga is the chanting of "ho ho" and "ha ha ha," which helps focus on the abdominal muscles and trains the diaphragm to allow one to laugh from the belly.

Change Your Breathing, Change Your Mind

There is a direct relationship between an individual's breathing pattern and his/her state of mind. When a person is stressed, breathing becomes fast, irregular and shallow. People tend to hold their breath if there are disturbing and negative thoughts in their minds. In contrast, when the mind is at peace, breathing is regular and deep.

Breathing is the only process that has a dual character. It continues automatically and is controlled by the unconscious mind, but it can also be consciously regulated. Through the practice of belly laughter and deep breathing, we can learn to change our breathing pattern from shallow to deep and easily alter our thoughts. Even if one is disturbed, deep breathing can help the body deal with stress better.

Laughter Yoga Connects People

Unconditional laughter connects people across cultures and countries no matter what language they speak or how they live. Laughter yoga promotes a strong union between those who laugh together, resulting in family-like bonds and a chance for providing social interaction and networking, which are essential for happiness. The goal of laughter yoga is to connect people without judgment, which is the true meaning of yoga.

Laughter Yoga Promotes Spiritual Growth

Laughter yoga goes beyond just laughing. Not only does it foster a feeling of physical well-being, it also enhances the spirit and touches the emotional core. It has the power to change one's state of mind from selfish to altruistic. It has been proved that people who laugh more are likely to be more generous and have more empathy than those who laugh rarely.

This inner spirit of laughter becomes apparent once people achieve a state of internal peace. The worries and intense goals that drive their lives become less important. They become aware that true happiness comes from giving unconditional love, sharing and caring for others. Laughter yoga inspires participants to make the world a better place not only for themselves but for everyone.

Scientific Rationale Behind Yoga and Laughter

According to yogic philosophy, the food we eat should be digested properly and the nutrients be well circulated in the body before being metabolized to produce energy. To do this, the body requires oxygen. To maintain good health, the digestive, circulatory and respiratory systems must be equally efficient.

Let us now examine how laughter yoga contributes to strengthening the body's functioning.

- **Toning the Digestive System:** The principal digestive organs like the stomach, intestines, liver and pancreas are situated in the abdominal cavity. They are supported by strong core muscles on all sides. The movement of the abdominal muscles and the diaphragm during respiration provides a gentle massage to these organs.

As part of laughter yoga, we perform different styles of belly laughter that exercise both the abdominal muscles and the diaphragm simultaneously. Scientists, in fact, refer to laughter as internal jogging that goes right into the belly and readjusts the internal organs. Regular laughter exercises not only strengthen the abdominal muscles but also hold the digestive organs in their place. This ensures proper digestion and absorption.

- **Strong Circulatory System:** The nutrients from the food we eat are absorbed into the blood. They are processed in the liver, passed on to the central pumping system and circulated in the body through a network of blood vessels. The blood also collects the wastes of metabolism and returns to the heart and lungs for purification.

The most important organ of circulation is the heart. Laughing promotes a healthy heart. A constant change in intra-thoracic pressure while laughing and breathing helps to draw in venous blood returning from the upper and lower parts of the body.

A good bout of laughter dilates the blood vessels. All of us have seen or experienced this as a flushed appearance and a feeling of warmth. As the circulatory system is stimulated, the pulse rate and blood pressure rise. In a nutshell, laughter helps tone the body's circulatory system.

- **Strengthened Respiratory System:** After the body tissues receive nutrients through the blood, they need oxygen to metabolize them. Laughter and breathing exercises help by increasing the capacity of the lungs and the net supply of oxygen to the body.

> **Dmitriy Efimov, Russia:** *I laughed every day for five months and lost ten pounds. This was excellent given that I do not follow a diet or play sports. Psychologically, too, a lot changed for me. I have begun to enjoy life again. Although I had everything to be happy, I could not bring myself to feel it. Now, everything has changed, I can express joy at every small thing, just like a child. Daily laughing has also improved my relationships with others. My friends, who find me smiling most of the time, are only too happy to smile in return.*

4

Laughter Yoga and
the Science of Breathing

*"Laughter and breathing bring you to the present as you
can't laugh and breathe in the past or future."*

I would practice yoga every day before the idea of laughter
clubs came to me. What I liked best about yoga was the
breathing exercise, or pranayama as it popularly called. It
made me feel energetic almost instantly. Though we treat
laughter as an exercise, we must study the physiology of
breathing to understand how laughter yoga, combined with
yogic breathing, allows more oxygen into our bodies and
brains.

Tidal Volume

Each lung holds a minimum of
3 liters of air in its resting state.
When we are not performing
any activity, we inhale and

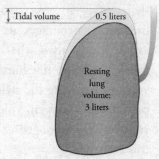

Tidal volume   0.5 liters

Resting
lung
volume:
3 liters

exhale about 500 milliliters (0.5 liters) of air with each breath. This average is called tidal volume.

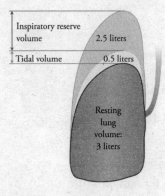

Inspiratory Reserve Volume

Our lungs are elastic. When we are engaged in a physical activity that demands more oxygen, the lungs can expand to inhale up to 2.5 liters of air. The medical term for this is inspiratory reserve volume.

Expiratory Reserve Volume

Out of the 3 liters of residual air that always stays in the lungs, we can force exhale about half—1.5 liters. This is called expiratory reserve volume. This residual air contains more carbon dioxide than oxygen. As yogic breathing encourages us to exhale longer than what we

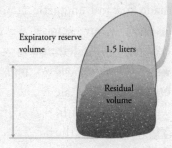

inhale, it helps the lungs to expel the expiratory reserve volume, replacing the stale air with fresh air that has a high percentage of oxygen. Voluntary laughter practice in laughter yoga is like prolonged exhalation, which helps to facilitate this exchange.

Vital Capacity

This is the sum of tidal volume, inspiratory reserve volume and expiratory reserve volume. In other words, it is a measurement of the maximum amount of air that you can breathe in and out in one cycle. When one is sedentary, many lung cells lie

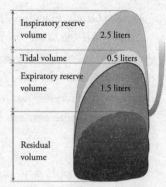

unused and become dysfunctional because they do not participate in the exchange of gases. The result is that even climbing stairs can cause shortness of breath. Laughter yoga offers a simple, easy and practical way for older adults, people with disabilities and others with a sedentary lifestyle to add some cardiovascular exercise to their routines.

It is important to understand that the body only has muscles of inhalation. Exhalation is passive and takes place when the lungs recoil. To force exhale extra air from the lungs, we need to use the abdominal muscles to push the diaphragm up. When we inhale to the maximum and keep laughing till we are out of breath, that state is called vital capacity laughter. It gives the lungs the best possible exercise by expanding them to their capacity.

When practiced over time, laughter yoga helps us to exhale double the amount of air than is inhaled. This means that laughter exercises can be compared to any other aerobic exercise that increases the heart rate and blood circulation and also improves oxygenation. This is why laughter exercises

Annelie Gareis, Ecuador: *I have been a daily laugher since May 2012. It has helped me lose weight without really changing my diet. Also, I have not fallen sick in five years. I feel more confident and happy, and I feel like I have grown spiritually. I believe the real benefits of laughter yoga came to me when I committed myself to practicing pranayama and laughter exercises every day.*

work well for people who don't get much exercise otherwise, especially senior citizens and physically challenged people. Laughing for as long as possible helps keep the lung cells healthy and uses the abdominal muscles even in the absence of strenuous physical workouts.

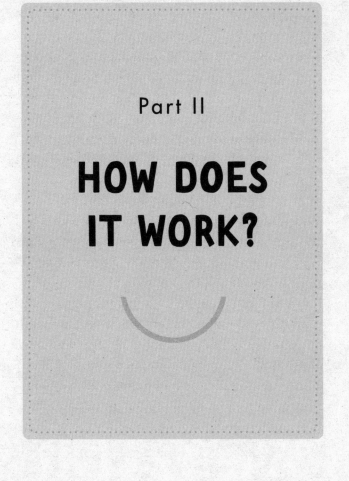

Part II

HOW DOES
IT WORK?

5

The Concept and Philosophy of Laughter Yoga

"We don't laugh because we are happy,
we are happy because we laugh."

—William James

Laughing for no reason is the core philosophy of laughter yoga. Traveling around the world, I am often asked: do we need a sense of humor to laugh? How can we laugh when we don't feel like laughing or are not in a good mood? How can we laugh when we have so many problems in life? Why can children laugh 300–400 times in a day while adults laugh less than fifteen times? Can we learn how to laugh?

Though I am a medical doctor, I must say I was not aware of these concerns when I started the laughter movement. But as the concept of laughter yoga evolved, so did the answers. I began to experience the magic of laughing without a reason, which gradually enabled me to discover the key concepts of the laughter yoga philosophy.

Developing a Sense of Humor Through Laughter

What is the relationship between sense of humor and laughter? Is it possible to laugh for no reason? Most people believe that one must have a sense of humor to be able to laugh, but laughter yoga has proved otherwise. No one is born with a sense of humor, which is the brain's capacity to perceive, relate to and experience a situation and judge if it is funny or not. We acquire this skill as our mental abilities develop. Sense of humor is essentially a mental and intellectual phenomenon.

Laughter, which arises from humor, is conditional. It depends upon an individual's intellectual ability, state of mind, level of happiness and satisfaction. However, laughter can be achieved unconditionally. Children laugh without any mental or cognitive ability to aid them in comprehending humor. Most of their laughter is an outcome of playfulness and inherent joy. To develop this ability to laugh joyfully, adults must let go of years of programmed behavior, layers of inhibition, conditioning and mental roadblocks created by themselves, their families and society. It is beneath these barriers that the infinite ability to laugh for no reason lies.

Teaching a person to develop a sense of humor is like flushing a blocked drain. Once the blockage is removed, the water starts to flow again. Similarly, mental inhibitions and shyness are like blockages to our sense of humor. Laughter yoga facilitates this flushing process by clearing out years of programmed behavior.

Laughter yoga techniques work even for those people who seem to have lost their ability to laugh or have absolutely no sense of humor. People often say, "I don't have a great sense of humor" or "I don't know any jokes." Somehow, people relate a sense of humor with the ability to tell jokes or do funny things. What we tell them at laughter clubs is: "It doesn't matter if you don't have a great sense of humor. Start laughing for no reason. It will help you widen your perception and develop a sense of humor."

Once released, natural laughter is hard to stop. In a country like India, where we don't have a great tradition of humor and comedy, hundreds of thousands of people laugh daily in public parks. People who never smiled now laugh at small things. They are able to tell jokes or act funny, something they never did before. By being playful, they have developed a sense of humor and brought more laughter into their lives.

Cause-and-Effect Relationship

Laughter and humor share a cause-and-effect relationship. They cannot be separated as one leads to the other. Sometimes humor is the cause, which is more mental and cognitive, while the effect is laughter, which is more of a physical phenomenon. In laughter yoga, laughter is the cause and humor is the effect. Through the laughter clubs and my travels to different parts of the world, I realized that most people do not identify with a sense of humor. They find it easier to laugh in a group. This is what led to the growing popularity of laughter yoga. So, even if you don't have a sense of humor, it does not matter. Just laugh for no reason and you will soon develop a funny bone.

Difference Between Laughter Yoga, Comedy Shows and Other Humor-Based Activities

People laugh during laughter yoga sessions, when they watch a comedy show and when they participate in any other humor-based activity. But first, let us understand the difference:

- Laughter yoga promotes laughter as a form of exercise along with breathing techniques based on yoga that bring about physiological and chemical changes that are conducive to good health. A comedy show, meanwhile, only amuses and entertains without focusing on health.
- In laughter yoga, every member gets to participate while in a comedy show the audience remains passive. It has been proved that people who actively participate in a laughter activity reap more health benefits than those who passively receive humor.
- In laughter yoga, the source of laughter is within the body and one can generate laughter with conscious effort and commitment whenever he/she wants to. On the other hand, laughing after watching a funny movie or comedy show has its source outside the body and is dependent on an external stimulus.
- Humor is subjective, while laughter is universal. When jokes are used to evoke laughter, chances are that many people may not like them or may find them to be

offensive. Laughter yoga minimizes, and even eliminates, this risk. When humor occurs during a laughter session, it is a spontaneous occurrence within the group. It is not forced, expected or required.

- During a laughter yoga session, it may take some people a while to open up and shed their inhibitions. But with time, their laughter gets better and they are able to laugh more. When people laugh at humorous situations and jokes, there is no certainty about how much they will laugh. In fact, people are likely to laugh less if they already know the punch lines.

- In a laughter yoga session, people can meet as often as the group wants without becoming boring. The members are encouraged to contribute creative inputs, such as inventing their own exercises, which keeps their interest and motivation high.

Theory of Motion Creates Emotion

How do you laugh when you're in no mood to, or when you don't feel like laughing? The answer is: theory of motion creates emotion.

There is an inherent connection between the body and the mind. Whatever happens to the mind happens to the body. If you observe sad and depressed people, their body language too appears similar. They walk slowly, talk slowly and their movements appear sluggish.

The opposite is also true. Whatever happens to the body happens to the mind. I remember my father saying, "If you are sad, don't sit idle. Keep doing something, or go for a walk and jog. You will feel better." He was right. I feel better when I stay active. This is what the theory of motion creating emotion is about. It establishes a two-way link between the body and the mind. If an individual changes the quality of thoughts, he/she will feel a change in body language. Conversely, if one brings about a change in body behavior, he/she will experience a change in mental state. Laughter yoga has the ability to synchronize both the body and the mind, thus maintaining harmony.

Two-Way Link Between Body and Mind

In 1884, psychologist William James found that one's state of mind, whether positive or negative, is mirrored by bodily expression, or body language. He found that each emotion triggers a corresponding behavior in the body and that enacting any emotion causes changes in an individual's state of mind.[1] The connection works both ways: from mind to body and body to mind.

Consider this:

- Sitting in a depressed posture and speaking in a dismal voice can lead to actual sadness.
- Actors who portray strong emotions often talk of real-life emotional repercussions. Many film and theater actors have reported feeling actual sadness while essaying tragic roles.
- Sexual thoughts lead to arousal of the sex organs while stimulation of the erogenous zones induces arousal in the mind.

The same phenomenon can be observed when it comes to athletes. Physically, they appear to be enthusiastic with their shouts and gestures, putting their minds into a positive state. This helps reduce fear and anxiety.

Soldiers use similar tactics when preparing for an attack and often shout at the top of their voices to psych themselves up. This bodily expression of courage triggers matching emotions in their minds.

Two Models of Laughter

- **Adult Model or Humor Model:** This is the mind–body model of laughter where our mind has to comprehend what is funny. For example, the extent to which a person laughs at a joke depends upon his/her ability to understand it, the quality of narration and his/her state of mind. This is because adults use cognitive ability to comprehend humor before laughing. But, the model has its limitations. It does not guarantee how much a person will laugh. It is conditional. It is dependent on sense of humor, state of mind and the quality of the external stimulus. For example, you will not laugh as much when you hear a joke for the second time.
- **Childlike Model or Body-Mind Model:** If you observe children, you will find that they laugh the most while playing. Children do not mull over what makes them laugh. They are not shy when it comes to laughing. This shows that the source of their laughter is within their bodies. Adults, too, can use the same

technique. A significant feature of this model is that the person must actively participate in laughter and humorous activities like playing games and singing or dancing in a group.

Fake It Until You Make It

There is an old saying, "If you are not happy, act like a happy person and you will become one." There is great wisdom and science behind "acting out happiness." According to the principles of Neuro-Linguistic Programming (NLP), there is hardly any difference between thinking about doing something and actually doing it. Hence, whatever may be the source of laughter, it leads to the same physiological changes in the body. This is reflected by what William James famously said: "We don't laugh because we are happy, we are happy because we laugh."

Difference Between Happiness and Joy

Laughter yoga marks a clear distinction between happiness and joy. Happiness is a conditional response that is dependent on the fulfillment of certain desires. It is related to circumstances that occurred in the past or may happen in the future and hardly deals with the present. Do you remember how long you were happy after completing a diploma, or getting a car, a job or a new house that you had worked for? Sadly, the fact is that even if all desired conditions are fulfilled, happiness is often fleeting as it is quickly displaced by new conditions—the idea of forever-moving goals.

In contrast, joy is unconditional commitment to being happy in the moment and to have fun despite all odds. It is easily triggered by activities such as laughing, dancing, singing and playing. Joy is a physical phenomenon while happiness is a state of mind.

When you are joyful, you experience physiological and biochemical changes due to the release of endorphins. Once you feel good, your perception of the world changes. In other words, joy is happiness from within that you can create on command and demand. Laughter yoga is all about learning to be joyful and navigating happiness in a better way.

Willingness and Commitment to Laugh

The most important factor in laughter yoga is the will of the participants to laugh. Laughter club members laugh voluntarily and with full commitment. This makes it easy for the group to laugh because when the mind is willing, anything is possible.

In contrast, when the mind is not ready to laugh, nobody can even make you smile. But why should you reserve laughter only for times when something funny or amusing happens? So often we leave laughter to chance rather than committing to joy. All that you need to do is to give yourself permission to laugh and nobody can stop you. You have to make an effort if you want to add more laughter to your life.

Childlike Play Is the Source of Laughter

Laughter is not just about laughing. It is about cultivating a childlike playfulness within oneself. Once you learn to play, you don't have to laugh. Laughter will become the natural outcome of your inner child. Though laughing in a group provides a stimulus, childlike behavior can help adults overcome inhibitions and loosen up. Therefore, laughter clubs incorporate many childlike actions such as producing funny sounds by swiveling the tongue inside the mouth, tapping cheeks filled with air, laughing like a child and talking gibberish.

As adults, very few people can retain the excitement of a child, which is why we continuously remind our members about its importance. Poems have been written about the desire to go back to one's childhood, but this alone is not enough. Some additional action is necessary. Just as one cannot learn how to swim without getting into the water, one has to behave like a child to be childlike. In laughter yoga, we revisit our childhood and try to carry over that carefree spirit to our daily lives.

The Difference Between Being Funny and Having Fun

An outsider looking at people doing laughter yoga and seeing them laugh for no reason may find it goofy and embarrassing. Most people are shy. They would rather laugh naturally instead of forcing it. If you ask laughter practitioners, they will tell you that they are totally into it and that there is nothing funny about it. According to them, it is all about having fun.

There is a difference between being funny and having fun. When one is being funny, he/she is performing in order to make others laugh. On the other hand, people participating in laughter exercises are not only making others laugh; they are making themselves laugh too.

A laughter session usually involves members playing like children. In fact, laughter is not just about the physical act of laughing; it is about also bringing out the inner child, which allows you to play as a grown-up. Once you learn to be playful, laughter becomes a natural outcome.

You Can Train Your Body and Mind to Laugh

Did you know that you can actually learn to laugh? Our bodies and minds can be trained to laugh at will. It's like learning to ride a bicycle, which uses muscle memory: once you learn it, you never forget. The NLP theory indicates that repeated bodily behavior over a period of time leads the mind to generate a predictable response. The body learns to produce a knee-jerk reaction without involving the process of thinking. This is called conditioning.

Russian scientist Ivan Pavlov's experiment with dogs is a classic example of conditioning. Every time he would give the dogs food, he would ring a bell. After several days of repeating this process, he stopped giving them food and only rang the bell. He found that simply ringing the bell, even in the absence of food, led the dogs to salivate and produce gastric juices. The dogs had developed an association between the ringing of the bell—a sensory experience—and food.

Similarly, the human brain can also be conditioned. With repetitive exercises, the body begins to react out of reflex before the brain can rationalize the response. Throughout our lives, we are conditioned by both positive and negative experiences that frame our personality.

NLP Conditioning with Laughter

When I started laughter yoga clubs in 1995, I did not have a philosophy in mind. It was later that I started looking into the science of NLP and found that the clubs had unconsciously incorporated many of its principles.

Our lives are nothing but a set of conditioned responses that develop as we grow up under the influence of people and events. For example, if you are expecting stressful phone calls from your workplace, over a period of time even the ringing of the phone can trigger stress. Even if it is someone wanting to share good news with you, your body will be hardwired to getting stressed.

According to the principles of NLP, we can program the body and mind for both good and bad experiences. This happens constantly in life and is known as conditioning. When we go through negative experiences like anxiety and fear, they are mostly the products of repeated past experiences. Here's an example: if you are afraid of your boss and he/she calls you to his/her office, your mind will immediately switch to negative thoughts. Your first reaction is likely to be, "Oh my god! What happened?"

If you have had several unpleasant experiences with him/her, even the sight of his/her car can elicit a negative bodily reaction. After a while, the conditioning is set so deep that just the sight of a similar car can make you feel anxious.

The body can also be programmed to respond positively. Laughter yoga allows one to cultivate feelings of joy and happiness. Each time we do a particular laughter exercise, we clap and chant "ho ho" and "ha ha ha." We repeat these exercises until they are wired into our nervous systems. You will be surprised to know that once this happens, you can feel happiness and joy just by clapping and chanting "ho ho" and "ha ha ha."

Another exercise we do during laughter yoga sessions is combining breathing and laughter. As part of this, the participants take a long deep breath with the instructor asking them to hold their breath and laugh as they exhale. After doing this repeatedly, laughter comes spontaneously the moment they breathe. I have personally experienced such conditioning. Several years ago I advised my participants to laugh while taking a shower. I decided to try it out for myself too. I started laughing in the shower every day, and soon this became a trigger for me. To this day, the moment I get into my bathroom I start laughing involuntarily. With laughter yoga, the brain develops new neuronal connections that trigger positive reactions in the body. These reactions lead the mind to experience the emotion of joy no matter what.

Over time, members of laughter clubs become conditioned to be joyful. Clapping in rhythm, chanting "ho ho" and "ha ha ha" in unison and using positive words like "very good" and "yay" are a few examples of the expressions of joy that are practiced at laughter clubs.

6

Voluntary vs. Real Laughter

"The more you laugh for no reason,
the more life will give you reasons to laugh."

Ever since I started conducting laughter yoga sessions, the most common criticism was that the laughter was forced and not genuine. Most people wondered if laughing this way was really beneficial or not. The question was whether the laughter in laughter yoga was real or not.

My answer is both yes and no. Yes, the sessions do begin with induced laughter, but it soon turns into genuine laughter. Even if we pretend to laugh, it leads to the same physiological and biochemical changes in the body as real laughter.

God has given mankind the ability to laugh—a gift not bestowed upon any other species. In fact, this extraordinary capability is inborn. Laughter is instinctive and almost everyone knows that there is just one way to laugh: when a funny situation arises. But laughter yoga has taught people to laugh without any reason.

Initially, jokes and comical anecdotes were used to make people laugh but this did not work for long. After some soul-searching it became clear that getting someone to make them laugh every day would not be feasible. That meant laughter had to be self-induced. There is no way that natural laughter can bring about physiological changes in the body as it is difficult to sustain.

It took some explanation and persuasion, but the participants finally agreed to give voluntary laughter a try. They were pleasantly surprised with the results. Psychologists say that the human mind tends to resist change, even if it is for the better. Similarly, I realized that anything new, particularly an idea such as laughing for no reason, would draw criticism. In fact, many onlookers felt that the laughter in laughter yoga was artificial and forced compared to the one arising from jokes, which they considered natural. According to them, artificial laughter could not possibly have any benefits. Considering this thought is wedged deep into people's minds, let me put the entire concept of "pretending to laugh" in perspective.

The Difference Between Real and Fake Laughter

Though laughter that results from jokes and laughter yoga are not the same, a closer look reveals more similarities than differences. The difference is only in the initial stage of providing a stimulus and triggering laughter. In one, a stimulus is provided and laughter is triggered by another person; in the other it is the person laughing who becomes the trigger.

In his book *Laughter: A Scientific Investigation*, Robert R. Provine says that one of the many things that make us laugh is laughter itself. He also says that we don't laugh a lot at funny or amusing things every day, but being around people creates more laughter opportunities. For example, we may laugh when we are with friends and say, "Hello! How are you?" even though the situation may not be funny.[1]

Mirror-Neuron Theory

As I observed people laughing in the laughter groups, I realized that not everyone laughed for the same reason. Some laughed only because the others were laughing. For instance, while watching a film in a theater, not everyone laughs because they understand a joke. Very often, the person next to you may laugh but still ask you what the joke was. He/she laughs because they see everyone around laughing. Putting it simply, we can say that laughter is contagious. In scientific terms, it is called the mirror-neuron theory.

Why do sports fans feel emotionally involved in the game and react as if they too are playing? Have you ever wondered why you end up eating when you see others eat even though you are not hungry? This ability to immediately comprehend what others are doing is an example of how this theory works.

The human brain has specialized cells called mirror neurons. It is due to these cells that we imitate and emulate the actions, behaviors and emotions of the people around us. Even if we are not learning actively, we unconsciously duplicate their actions. This is why we are called products of our environment. A person is known by the company he/she keeps. If you are among good people, you will copy their positive traits, but if you are among grumpy people, you are likely to become like them. You can blame it on the mirror neurons.

In the early 1990s, Italian neuroscientist Giacomo Rizzolatti, who works at the University of Parma, accidentally discovered the existence of mirror neurons in the brains of monkeys. This happened when, sitting in front of a monkey, a scientist picked up something to eat. Rizzolatti immediately noticed the stimulation of cells in the motor area of the monkey's brain. This stimulation was linked to a hand movement similar to the scientist's. Though the monkey did not move, there was a stimulation of brain cells that projected a similar movement. This led Rizzolatti to conclude that it is not only the physical actions we copy; we even mirror the emotions of other people. This, in fact, is the basis for communication and empathy.[2]

I found that people could easily learn to laugh because of the presence of these neurons. They could copy the actions and behavior of others who were joyful and happy without a reason. Therefore, thanks to mirror neurons, members of laughter clubs are not only good at imitating the emotions of laughter, joy and happiness, but are also very good at replicating virtues of compassion, love, appreciation and forgiveness.

Fake Laughter Is Good

The genesis of this concept is based on scientific studies that say that real and intentional laughter offer the same benefits.

As a medical doctor, I understood that voluntary laughter would have similar cardiovascular and respiratory demands as spontaneous laughter. Whether you are laughing at a joke or pretending to laugh, you are exhaling stale air and inhaling oxygen. This exchange of gases is what matters because as long as the body gets oxygen, how you laugh is not important. Today, several scientific studies conducted across the world have proved that the benefits of laughter yoga are real, even if the laughter is not.

U.S. Study on Forced Laughter

Psychologists say that just a minute of forced laughter can help beat the blues. "Forced laughter is a powerful, readily available and cost-free way for many adults to regularly boost their mood and psychological well-being," said Charles E. Schaefer, professor of psychology at Fairleigh Dickinson University in Teaneck, New Jersey.[3]

His findings come from two experiments conducted on thirty-nine college students and Teaneck residents. While studies involving larger samples are needed to bolster his conclusions, Professor Schaefer said that these initial results were important enough to warrant attention. He also discovered the salubrious effect of artificial laughter in a study involving seventeen Fairleigh Dickinson students. He first asked them questions to gauge their mood. Then he directed them to laugh heartily for a minute and tested them again. On an average, the subjects reported feeling significantly better after sixty seconds of fake laughter.

Why does fake laughter work? This happens because your body doesn't know it is fake even though your brain might. Professor Schaefer said, "Once the brain signals the body to laugh, the body doesn't care why. It's going to release endorphins; it's going to relieve stress as a natural physiological response to the physical act of laughing."

Professor Schaefer also designed a second study to compare the effects of forced laughter with that of continuous smiling and howling. He directed twenty-two participants to smile broadly for sixty seconds, then laugh heartily for sixty seconds and finally howl for the same duration. He found that while both laughing and smiling helped boost spirits, howling did not. Forced laughter proved to be the most beneficial of the three. "One minute of forced laughing showed a significantly greater improvement than one minute of smiling," he concluded.

Converting Voluntary Laughter into Genuine Giggles

The growing popularity of laughter yoga indicates that people are deriving health benefits from it. Laughter yoga is based not just on theory but also on practical experience. Laughter is derived from the body, not from the mind. It is the result of cultivating childlike playfulness: a very difficult quality to develop as an adult. Laughter clubs provide an ideal platform to develop a playful attitude and help people laugh more than they normally would. They encourage members to participate in a number of playful techniques that help convert self-induced laughter into real laughter.

Acting Happy

Paul Ekman and Robert Levenson, psychologists from the University of California, have arrived at the conclusion that the advice to "put on a happy face" may actually be beneficial. Their research shows that facial expressions are not only reactions to emotional states but can also provoke these states. The latter is what happens in laughter yoga.[4]

Could acting be the next transformational health trend? You can actually change your personality just by acting the way you want to be. Tom Cruise has rescued people in real life on more than five occasions, thanks to having acted bravely in movies. Performing sadness can make you depressed, too. Many actors have slipped into depression after playing sad roles for a long time. The social psychologist Amy Cuddy popularized a new practice of power posing, according to which just changing your posture can help you become more confident. Psychologist Dr. Robert Epstein found that some movie stars who go through the motions of being lovers during rehearsals have actually fallen in love and have become real-life partners. In India, arranged marriages are very common, and couples who start practicing loving behavior after they are married eventually become soul mates.

Our bodies play a very important role in shaping our thoughts. George Lakoff, a former professor at the University of California, Berkeley, and pioneer in embodied cognition, says that changing our body's behavior can change our thoughts. Our minds are very complicated, but our bodies are easier to comprehend. We can reverse engineer our emotions by using the body-mind connection.

Laughter Yoga Activates Laughter Muscles

Yogic laughter exercise is not a substitute for the spontaneous laughter that we may experience through the day. However, it does help to increase our capacity to laugh. According to other research, if you stretch your laughter muscles on a regular basis, they will respond more spontaneously whenever there is something amusing. Laughing on a daily basis exercises the facial muscles and increases the muscle tone, which helps to maintain a smile.

There is no need to judge the quality of laughter as you will enjoy benefits from both voluntary and spontaneous laughter. If you observe a typical laughter yoga session, the initial warm-up exercises ultimately lead to genuine laughter. In fact, several scientific studies have come out in support of laughter yoga and its methods.

7

Fifteen Steps of
Laughter Yoga in a Group

"Laughter is too important to be left to chance.
Make a commitment toward it and go for it."

You will be able to enjoy the benefits of laughter only if you actually laugh. We already know from scientific research that even voluntary laughter impacts physiology and biochemistry. All you need to do is to gather a group of people and do the laughter exercises together. Normally, ten to fifteen people make for a good group, but you can also try with five to ten people.

Laughter yoga sessions are structured programs where someone has to lead and give step-by-step instructions to the group.

Duration

The fifteen steps that are a part of a typical laughter session, including popular laughter exercises, usually take about twenty minutes. You can find a list of more exercises in the appendix, as you don't have to do the same exercises each time. Keep trying new ones and create your own.

Basic Rules to Follow During a Laughter Yoga Session

- You will get the benefits of laughter even if you laugh intentionally. Faking laughter is fine.
- When laughing in a group, one should keep moving around and meeting the others and maintain eye contact. This will lead to real and contagious laughter.
- Do not overexert or apply too much force while laughing. Try to be playful. Less force translates into more enjoyment.
- Since we do voluntary laughter exercises, try to laugh for longer in order to get rid of the residual air in your lungs. Each laughter exercise lasts between thirty seconds and one minute. However, there are no hard-and-fast rules. You can keep laughing as long as the group is enjoying it.
- Laughter exercises should be interspersed with deep-breathing exercises as described below.

Clapping and Warm-up Exercises

Since it is not easy to laugh without a reason, laughter sessions start with warm-up exercises such as clapping and chanting "ho ho" and "ha ha ha" (refer to pictures on the following page). This reduces inhibitions and makes it easier for people to laugh. Also, we clap with our hands parallel to each other for full finger-to-finger and palm-to-palm contact. This stimulates acupressure points in the hands and increases energy levels. Later, we add rhythm to the clapping to further boost energy levels and group synchronicity. The rhythm that is often followed is 1–2, 1–2–3.

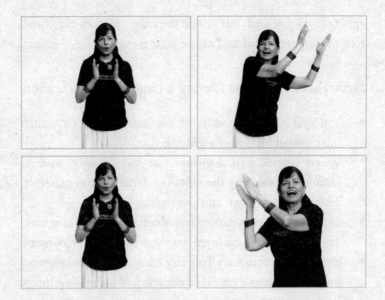

Chanting and Moving

We add a simple chant to clapping like "ho ho" and "ha ha ha." These are heavy exhalations that come from the belly and stimulate the diaphragm. While moving, smile and maintain eye contact with the others in the group. Enthusiastic clapping and chanting helps build positive energy, gets the diaphragm moving and creates a group dynamic that prepares you for laughter.

Deep-Breathing Exercises

Laughter exercises are interspersed with deep-breathing exercises to help flush the lungs and aid physical and mental relaxation.

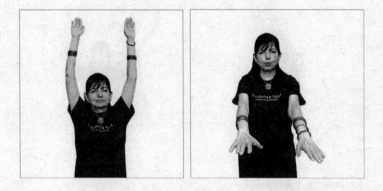

From a relaxed standing position, bend forward at the waist to a point where you are comfortable (different for everyone) while exhaling through the mouth. Let your arms dangle and relax. Stand up straight while inhaling through your nose and taking as deep a breath as possible. Lift your arms up, slightly stretching your body backward. Hold your breath for four to five seconds. Exhale slowly as you bring your arms down and bend forward. Repeat this twice (refer to the pictures above).

Childlike Playfulness

One of the objectives of laughter yoga is to cultivate childlike playfulness. We have special childlike cheers such as "very good (clap), very good (clap), yay" to encourage the group. You can do this by swinging your arms upward with childish exuberance. In between laughter and breathing exercises, the entire group keeps chanting "very good, very good, yay" (refer to the pictures on the following page).

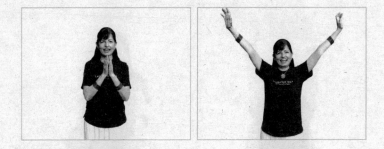

Greeting Laughter

- **Namaste Laughter:** Since laughter yoga originated in India, the first exercise is to greet everyone around you by joining both hands, looking into their eyes and laughing.
- **Handshake Laughter:** You may also shake hands with the other members of your group and laugh. You can also combine namaste laughter and handshake laughter.

To end the laughter exercises, start clapping and chanting "ho ho" and "ha ha ha" three to four times, followed by "very good, very good, yay." In fact, all exercises should end with these chants. You can also try the following exercises.

- **Milkshake Laughter:** Hold two imaginary glasses of milk or any other drink in your hands. Pretend to pour milk from one glass into another while chanting "aayaayyy." Then pretend to pour it back into the first glass saying "aayaayyy." After this, everyone laughs and pretends to drink from the glass (refer to pictures on the following page). This process is to be repeated thrice, followed by claps and chants of "ho ho" and "ha ha ha." If you don't like milk, you can pretend to throw it behind you or on the ground in front of you.

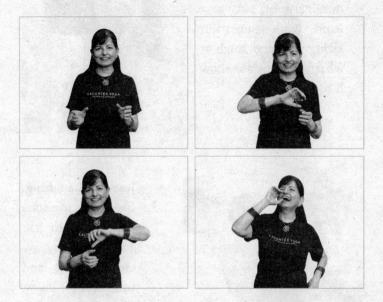

- **Cell Phone Laughter:** Imagine your cell phone rings. Put it to your ear and laugh as if you have heard the funniest joke ever. Move around and share it with the others, laughing all the while. You can also pretend to hold two imaginary 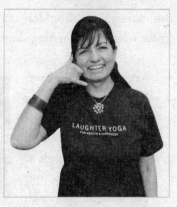 phones in both your hands and laugh into them in turn.

- **Credit Card Bill Laughter:** Hold an imaginary bill in your hand (with the palm facing you) and laugh at what you see. Also show it to the others.

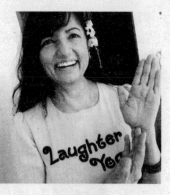

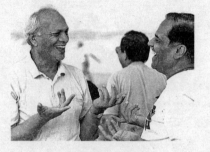

- **Just Laughing:** Imagine someone coming up to you and asking why you are laughing and you don't know. Hold your palms out, shrug your shoulders and pretend as if to say, "I don't know why I am laughing, I am just laughing."

- **Argument Laughter:** Point your finger at the other members of the group, pretending to argue and laugh at the same time. You can also do this with

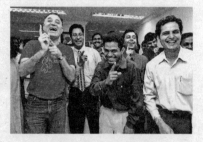

two groups facing each other and laughing competitively, pretending to argue.

- **Lion Laughter:** This laughter has been derived from the yogic posture called *simha* mudra (lion posture). Stick your tongue out while keeping your mouth and eyes 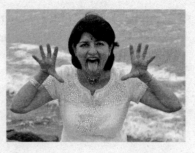 wide open. Hold your hands out like a lion's paws and roar. Lion laughter is a very good exercise to get rid of inhibitions and exercise the facial muscles, tongue and the throat. It also improves blood supply to the thyroid gland.

- **Silent Laughter with the Mouth Wide Open:** Keep your mouth wide open and laugh without making any sound. Laugh gently without applying too much force. Look into the eyes of the other group members to ensure that the laughter is contagious.

- **Gradient Laughter:** This laughter is practiced at the end of a session. All the members are asked to come closer to the leader. This exercise starts by smiling and looking at each other. Gradually, the leader introduces gentle giggles, which the others follow. The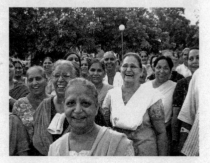

intensity of laughter is increased gradually with all the members bursting into hearty laughter for about a minute.

- **One-Yard Laughter:** This laughter exercise mimics how we measure a yard using our hands. You can do this by stretching one arm out to the side, moving the other one over it and bringing it back to the shoulder. The movement resembles that of an archer preparing to shoot. The arm itself moves in three jerks with chants of "aayaay, aayaay, aayaay." After this, the participants burst into laughter by stretching both their arms to the side and throwing their heads back a little. The imaginary measuring of a yard begins from the left side. This cycle is to be repeated twice (refer to the pictures below).

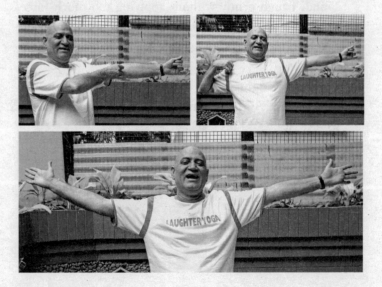

- **Hot Soup Laughter:** Stick your tongue out and move your wrists up and down, pretending to cool your mouth down after taking a sip of very hot soup. Keep laughing as you do this.

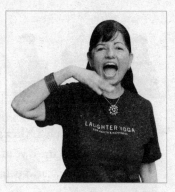

- **Electric Shock Laughter:** Reach out to the other members of the group as if to shake hands. Pretend that you got an electric shock from the touch. Laugh at the surprise.

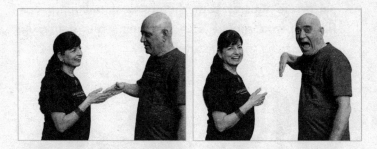

Ten Laughter Exercises for Couples

- **High Five/High Ten Laughter:** Stand facing your partner and give them a high five (slap your right palm against your partner's right palm and then repeat the movement with your left hand). Now, do this with both your hands to give your partner a high ten. Keep laughing and alternate between high fives and high tens (refer to the pictures on the following page).

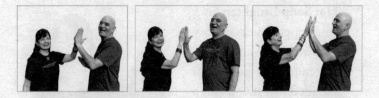

- **Look into Each Other's Eyes and Try Not to Laugh:** Keep looking into your partner's eyes and try not to laugh. Put on a serious face and see who laughs first.

- **Milking the Cow Laughter:** Intertwine the fingers on both your hands and turn them toward the ground, making your thumbs look like a cow's teats. Ask your partner to squeeze your thumbs as if milking a cow. Both of you should keep laughing while doing this exercise (refer to the pictures below).

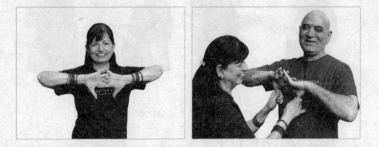

- **Peek-a-Boo Laughter:** Both partners must cover their faces with their hands and then remove them as if playing peek-a-boo. Keep laughing as you do this (refer to the pictures on the following page).

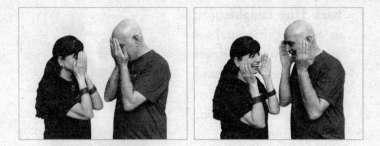

- **Remote Control Laughter:** One person starts to laugh as the other pretends to press the ON button on an imaginary remote control. Then he/she presses the OFF button, which is a signal for their partner to stop laughing. Repeat the action and laugh (refer to the pictures below).

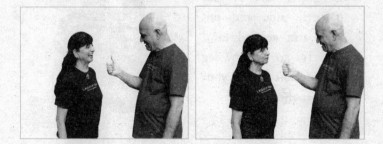

- **Selfie Laughter:** Pretend to take a selfie with your partner by holding your palm up like a cell phone. Keep laughing and taking pictures.

- **Hugging Laughter:** Hug your partner and keep laughing to feel each other's laughter vibrate in your own body.

- **Back Hug Laughter:** Sit or stand with your back touching your partner's back and lock your elbows together. Laugh and feel the laughter vibrating through your body.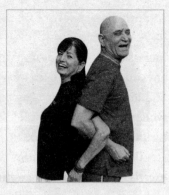

- **Follow the Leader:** One partner pretends to be the leader and starts making different laughter sounds. The other partner has to mimic these sounds.

- **Standing on One Leg Laughter:** Stand by your partner's side and put your arm around him/her. Try to lift the leg that doesn't touch your partner and laugh.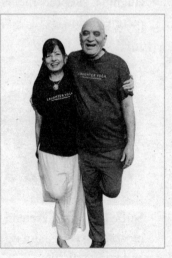

Who Should Not Do Laughter Yoga Exercises?

Laughter yoga is not a miracle cure and should not be treated as a substitute for medical consultation for physical, mental and psychological illnesses. It is a powerful and natural complementary form of healing, but it may not be suitable for everyone as it involves some physical strain and an increase in intra-abdominal pressure. Laughter yoga is like any other aerobic exercise to which all precautions apply. Should you experience any discomfort, pain or breathlessness while doing the laughter exercises, please discontinue and seek medical advice.

People suffering from the following ailments should exercise caution and consult a doctor before joining a laughter club: hernia, advanced piles (hemorrhoids), heart diseases with chest pain, epilepsy, severe backache and utero-vaginal prolapse. Also, women who are pregnant and those who have recently undergone surgery must proceed with caution.

Minor Discomfort after Laughter Yoga

- **Heaviness in the Head or Mild Headache:** Some people complain about their head feeling heavy or of mild to moderate headaches after doing laughter yoga exercises. This happens occasionally and is usually not a cause for concern. It may happen due to excessive force being applied while doing the laughter exercises. Take it easy the next time. Other reasons for headaches after doing laughter yoga exercises are high blood pressure and chronic migraines. People looking to do these exercises must get their blood pressure checked if they are on the borderline or have hypertension.
- **Throat Irritation:** Another common complaint is irritation of the throat or mild cough. Don't get worried about this and laugh softly the next time.

8

Laughter Meditation

"The most wasted of all days is that
on which one has not laughed."

—Nicolas Chamfort

When we do laughter yoga exercises, we have to make an effort to laugh. But when we are part of a group, the laughter becomes spontaneous and effortless. It flows like a fountain. This is the state of laughter meditation. Once you reach this point, you don't laugh; you become laughter. It is this deeper experience of unconditional laughter that is different from laughter exercises. Laughter meditation is the purest kind of laughter and a very cathartic experience that opens up the subconscious mind, allowing one to experience laughter from deep within.

Laughter meditation requires one to make a conscious effort to stay detached from mental, emotional and physical distractions. While laughing, we do not have any conscious thoughts and all our senses naturally and effortlessly combine to give us joy, peace and relaxation.

Laughter as Dynamic Meditation

There are two broad categories of meditation: still and dynamic. When you focus on and get involved in an activity or movement it becomes dynamic meditation. Since you are not thinking of anything else, you start enjoying the activity. Some examples of dynamic meditation are chanting mantras, singing, dancing, playing and laughing. Another example is that of children not being mindful of the world while playing.

One of the reasons why people fail to meditate is because they cannot control their thoughts. The moment they try to meditate, thoughts start flowing into their minds and they give up. They think that it is difficult as they cannot get rid of their thoughts. Since the mind's behavior is not still but dynamic, it is better to start with dynamic meditation. You can move on to still meditation once the mind is more focused.

Initially, laughter meditation should be practiced in a group, which makes it easier to experience the wisdom of laughing without a reason. Once you have mastered it, you can practice laughter meditation all by yourself. If you are a first-timer, I suggest that you try doing the exercises in small groups with family members or friends. Start by sitting in a circle so that everyone can see each other. Laugh slowly as in gradient laughter and gradually increase the intensity. Initially, you may find it absurd to laugh without a reason, but eventually group dynamics and the infectious nature of laughter will help you laugh for real.

Laughter as Catharsis

People often start crying during laughter meditation. This is because laughter helps to release pent-up feelings and emotions stored in the subconscious mind. Therefore, laughter is both a physical as well as a psychological release. It also helps to release anger and frustration. As a result, people are more calm than before when dealing with everyday problems. It also helps them be less judgmental.

Guidelines to Achieving a Meditative State of Laughter

- **Duration:** Group laughter meditation can be done for ten to twenty minutes. Do it for ten minutes in a sitting position with your eyes open and then take a short break of five minutes. After this, lie down with your eyes closed and laugh for another ten minutes.
- **Ideal Venue:** The indoors are well-suited for laughter meditation as there are minimum distractions. While selecting a venue, ensure that it is comfortable, clean and peaceful. You can also use yoga mats.
- **How to Sit:** You should sit in a relaxed position on the floor with your legs folded and eyes open so that you can see others laughing. You can also let your body move naturally while laughing. Ensure that you sit in a circle so that everyone can see each other and maintain eye contact.
- **No Talking, No Distractions:** The most important thing to remember is that nobody must talk or try to communicate in any way (no winks, funny faces or

sounds) as that will engage the conscious mind instead of allowing it a release.

How to Go About Laughter Meditation?

It is best to begin with some warm-up laughter exercises. This will energize the group members and help them get rid of their inhibitions.

- Place your hands in front of your chest with the palms facing outward. Push them forward twice saying "ho ho" aggressively. After this, push your palms down twice and chant "ha ha ha" to stimulate the diaphragm. Take a few deep breaths and repeat. Alternatively, you can begin with gradient laughter where people start by laughing softly and gradually increase the intensity. Soon, it becomes infectious and sets off a chain reaction.

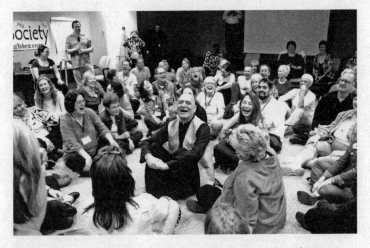

Dr. Madan Kataria during a laughter meditation session in Chicago.

- When you sit in a group and watch the others laugh, laughter flows spontaneously and effortlessly. The key factor here is eye contact.

- Do laughter meditation for about five minutes. Then take a few deep breaths and observe a minute of silence.

- After one minute, start laughing softly and gradually build the group laughter for another five minutes.

- Next, lie down on the floor, close your eyes and allow the laughter to build up. This can be done for five to ten minutes, after which everyone should take a few deep breaths. Observe silence and relax the body.

- End with yoga *nidra* relaxation, which is discussed in the next chapter.

9

Yoga Nidra in Laughter Yoga

"Seven days without laughter makes one weak."

—Mort Walker

Yoga nidra means yogic sleep where the mind is conscious and awake but the body goes to sleep. Sleep is a natural recharge mechanism for the body and mind. In today's stressful times, many people do not get enough sleep. They feel drowsy through the day and cannot focus or concentrate. Consequently, efficiency and performance drop.

Yoga nidra is a powerful relaxation technique that helps the body recharge quickly so that you can perform to the maximum. Just thirty minutes of yoga nidra will offer relaxation equivalent to two hours of ordinary sleep. If you don't get enough time to sleep at night, do yoga nidra any time during the day to feel refreshed.

Laughter is a dynamic energy that helps to energize every cell in the body. It also releases a lot of emotions from the subconscious mind, especially when we do laughter meditation after the exercises. Therefore, we need some grounding techniques in place to ensure that the physiology of the body is normal. Like with any other exercise, the body needs to relax at the end of a laughter yoga session too.

Mind Programming Technique

We often struggle to give up bad habits but are unable to do so despite our best efforts. We end up with new resolutions that are hard to implement. This is because we make these decisions using our conscious mind without making changes to our subconscious or deeper mind.

Yoga nidra helps you connect with your subconscious mind. Whatever you say or hear while doing yoga nidra is registered into your subconscious mind. If you want to change your lifestyle or a habit, all you need to do is make a resolution and say it thrice before starting yoga nidra and at the end. Yoga nidra, which opens up the subconscious mind, helps the change to manifest effectively. For example, if your resolution is to exercise regularly, just say, "I'm doing my morning exercises daily." Repeat this thrice before and after you do yoga nidra. It is important that the resolution be in the present tense and not in the future. Always say, "I am doing ..." instead of "I will do ..."

Gateway to Meditation

It is very difficult for most of us to meditate because there is a continuous stream of thoughts that keeps coming even if we try to stop it. Our mind cannot concentrate unless the body is relaxed. Therefore, the first step to meditation is to relax the body. Yoga nidra provides the easiest way to do so and help you focus, thereby leading to a meditative state.

Anyone Can Do It

Yoga nidra is suitable for everyone regardless of age. All you have to do is lie down on the floor or sit on a chair. The technique is so simple that you cannot go wrong. Just follow the instructions of the facilitator. It is likely that you may fall asleep, but you will still reap the benefits as the unconscious mind absorbs the practice. Essentially, it is simple meditation that controls thoughts. You can practice it for anywhere between five minutes and one hour.

There are many standard yoga nidra audios available for download on cell phones. Alternatively, you can record the steps and play them, or have someone else read the instructions out to you while you lie down and follow them. Once you have memorized the steps, you can instruct yourself silently.

Step-by-Step Instructions

- **Preparing for Yoga Nidra**

a) Lie down on your back and be comfortable. Put your hands by your sides with the palms facing upward. Maintain a little distance between your feet.

b) It is important to remain still throughout the session. As far as possible, try not to move your body. Occasional movement is fine.

c) Take a few deep breaths and let your body relax. Feel your belly rise and fall as you inhale and exhale. With each exhalation, relax all the muscles and try coinciding exhalation with relaxation. Take slower, longer and deeper breaths and repeat five times.

- **Making a Resolution**

If you wish to bring about a change in your habits or improve your lifestyle, say it in your mind thrice. You can also visualize your resolution in your mind.

- **Body Scan or Moving Awareness**

a) Move awareness to different parts of your body. Visualize and focus on specific body parts: forehead, eyebrows, the muscles around your eyeballs, right cheek, left cheek, bridge of the nose, upper lip, lower lip, chin, jaw muscles, tongue, the back of the head, the back of the neck, shoulders, upper arm, elbows, forearms, hands, chest, abdominal muscles, pelvic muscles, upper back, lower back, buttocks, thighs, knee joints, calf muscles and the feet. Feel them relax.

b) Imagine a wave of relaxation passing through your body. Feel it as it passes from the head and makes its way to the toes.

c) Focus on your right hand, thumb, index finger, middle finger, ring finger, little finger, palm, wrist, forearm, elbow, upper arm, right shoulder, the right side of your chest, the right side of your abdomen, the right thigh muscles, the right knee joint, the right calf muscles, the right ankle and the right foot and its toes. Repeat the sequence for your left side.

• **Breath awareness**

Turn your attention to how you breathe.

a) Start observing how you breathe and focus on the nose and the upper lip.

b) Feel the cool air touching the inside of your nose when you inhale and the warm air on your upper lip when you exhale. Turn your attention to how you breathe, follow your breath from the beginning to the end.

c) Focus on your chest and become aware of its movement. Feel your chest expanding when you inhale and returning to normal when you exhale.

d) Feel the movement in your abdomen as you breathe. Take a slow, deep breath. Feel your belly rise when you inhale and fall when you exhale. Make your breathing slower, longer and deeper. Try coinciding exhalation with relaxation of all the muscles in your body. With each exhalation, tell yourself that you are 10 percent more relaxed than the previous breath. Repeat this five times.

e) Now imagine that you are breathing into the entire body. Take a slow, long and deep breath. Keep breathing slowly and try to coincide relaxation with exhalation.

• **Visualization**

Using your imagination, try to visualize, as if you are watching a movie. Try to see movement, colors and sound in what you visualize. If you don't see anything, relax and be patient but don't force it. Allow yourself to see whatever your mind pictures without any judgment or analysis. You may select some of the following visualizations depending on how much time you have.

a) Imagine a sunrise behind the mountains.
b) Imagine a group of white birds flying in the early morning sky.
c) Imagine taking a walk on the beach and feeling the cool air on your face.
d) Imagine sitting on the beach with your eyes closed. Hear the waves coming in and going out.
e) Feel the sand under your feet as you walk on the beach.
f) Imagine the smell of the sea and the sound of the seagulls. Hear the other birds chirping early in the morning.
g) Imagine sitting in a boat with your hands in the water. Feel the coolness of the water as it touches your hands and legs.
h) Imagine walking on the grass. Feel the dew under your feet.
i) Imagine you are in the woods. Feel the touch of the earth against your body.

• **Opposite Sense Perceptions**

Let's move through a series of opposite sensations that will allow you to experience a range of perceptions.

a) Imagine feeling very cold. Feel yourself shivering. Next, imagine feeling extremely hot and sweating because of the intense heat. Feel your body becoming hotter. Now, relax and return to normal.

b) Feel your presence becoming bigger. Imagine your body becoming the size of a giant, as if resembling a big building. Once you feel your body has reached its peak, restrain your energy and begin to contract. Imagine your body becoming smaller, and feel yourself shrink to a point where it can fit into the smallest of containers.

c) Imagine lying on the floor. Feel the ground against your body. Feel your body becoming heavier. Imagine all the stresses and tensions melting away into the ground. Feel your body becoming light and relaxed. Feel it becoming weightless. Return to normal and take a few deep abdominal breaths.

• **Repeat the Resolution**

Repeat the resolution you made in the beginning thrice or imagine seeing pictures of what you wish to create for yourself. Feel as if it is already happening and that you are living your dream.

• **Return to Normal**

a) Start becoming aware of your breathing. Inhale into the whole of your body and relax. Imagine that the breaths you are taking are not only going into your lungs but also to each and every cell of your body. Repeat this five times. Begin a countdown from ten and wake up slowly.

b) Start moving your fingers and toes.

c) Slowly take a long, deep breath and stretch.
d) Rub your palms gently.
e) Place your hands over your eyes.
f) Turn to one side and sit up gently.

- **Voice Command Instructions**

a) The voice should be tender and soft.
b) When giving instructions, be simple and direct.
c) Ensure the voice is calm and paced with regular pauses.
d) You can speak like this: "Bring your attention to …" or "Re … lax" or "… 5, 4, 3, 2, 1." Allow the sound to move through your body as you stretch the words.

Part III

LEARNING TO LAUGH MORE

10

Cultivating the Habit of Smiling

"A smile is a curve that sets everything straight."

—Phyllis Diller

A smile is the first non-verbal language we learn. In fact, smiling has been in use for centuries to communicate feelings of warmth. A very effective tool, it can make you and everyone around you feel good. It is also a safe way to communicate with strangers.

There are three types of smiles: intentional, spontaneous and inner smile.

Intentional Smile

This smile can be particularly effective at the workplace, where you may be required to smile even when you don't want to. I have observed that 80 to 90 percent of people return a smile even if we don't know them. This fake intentional smile brings about physiological reactions that elevate the mood and make one feel happier, lighter and better. Intentional smiling is also a good coping tool when dealing with stressful and anxiety-laden situations.

Spontaneous Smile

This is a genuine, feel-good response to something positive, be it seeing an old friend, hearing some good news, watching your children play or hearing and seeing something funny. The corners of the mouth are turned up, but the stimulus for that response is not strong enough to trigger hearty laughter.

Inner Smile

This is a positive reflection of your inner being that stays on the face for as long as the positive feelings stay. This kind of a smile can often be seen on the faces of truly spiritual and happy people who float on a cloud of bliss most of the time.

How to Maintain a Smile on Your Face

Exercising your facial muscles by laughing and smiling on a regular basis tones the smiling muscles and keeps the face prepared to smile more. The act of smiling has a lot to do with basic body movements—the more we exercise the muscles required to smile, the more we end up smiling. This phenomenon is based on the theory of motion creates emotion. If you are physically active, exercise regularly and engage in a sport or dancing, you are likely to smile and laugh more.

The Duchenne Smile

This smile activates the part of the brain responsible for happiness. The Duchenne smile is named after French neurologist Guillaume Benjamin Amand Duchenne, who experimented with and studied the muscles of the face when a person was smiling. He discovered that when the lips part and turn up, and the eyes crinkle, the upper lip droops slightly and there is heightened activity in the left anterior region of the cortex, which is the center for happy emotions. Even an induced smile can help a gloomy person feel upbeat.

I have personally benefited from the Duchenne smile. In the beginning, when I would laugh without involving my eye muscles, I did not feel so great. But after learning about the involvement of these muscles, I consciously started to crinkle my eyes while laughing. And yes, I felt the difference. My laughter was more enjoyable and relaxing. It also brought about a significant change in my mood.

How Laughter Yoga Keeps You Smiling

Not only is laughter yoga a powerful tool for boosting personal development and self-confidence but it also tones the facial muscles and brings a smile to your face. It creates a safe environment for others to connect with you, which goes a long way to achieving success in all aspects of life: professional, personal and social. A genuine smile is the index of your happiness, so put a little more joy into your smile, reach out to others and give a little more of yourself when you smile next.

German Study on Holding Chopsticks Between the Teeth: Mimicking a Smile

A study conducted by four German scientists has shown that various facial expressions lead to different changes in the brain, which influence performance and behavior. This significant research is important for all laughter professionals as it reaffirms a core teaching of laughter yoga—that our body cannot differentiate between real and fake laughter. It restates the fact that laughter originating from the body can trigger changes in our brain and generate real emotions.

The study in question asked the participants to hold chopsticks between their teeth, which induced a smile by contracting a particular group of muscles. This led to a release of dopaminergic chemicals that regulated mood.

Three groups were studied. The first group held the chopsticks horizontally between their teeth (this resembled a smile). The second held it vertically between the lips while the third group got no chopsticks.

The study concluded that inducing facial expressions does lead to release of neurochemicals that ensure a positive mood and boost the sense of well-being. It confirms that faking a smile too brings about positive changes in the brain. This logically follows that laughing with your whole body, as practiced in laughter yoga, must be sending a lot of powerful biofeedback to the brain cells.[1]

Practical Ideas to Smile More Every Day

- **Strengthen Your Smile Muscles:** There are three muscles that help us smile: orbicularis oculi (around the eyes), zygomaticus major (elevates the corners of your mouth) and orbicularis oris (the muscles of your lips). The best way to exercise these muscles is to stand in front of a mirror and smile. Part your lips and raise the corners of your mouth as in an ear-to-ear grin. Finally, crinkle your eyes and maintain this smile for five to ten seconds. Repeat five times every day.

- **Smiling at Strangers:** Smile at five strangers every day and see how many smile back. I bet the result will be 99 percent!

- **Using Chopsticks to Smile:** Whenever you are angry, upset or stressed out, place a pencil or chopsticks between your teeth for a few minutes. Keep looking at yourself in the mirror and try to vocalize the sound of "he he he." The contraction of your facial muscles will lead to happy chemicals being produced in your brain and will definitely change your state of mind.

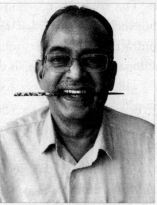

- **Combine Breathing with Your Smile:** Take a deep breath and smile. Maintain this for five seconds and return to normal while exhaling. Repeat five to ten times.

- **Smile with Your Eyes:** Stand in front of a mirror, cover your mouth and nose with your hands and try to smile using your eyes.

- **Visualize Yourself Smiling:** Close your eyes and visualize yourself smiling. Do this for five to ten seconds.

11

Practice Laughter Yoga Alone

"Know laughter, do laughter, be laughter."

If you want to pursue a master's degree in laughter, learn to laugh alone. This is the best thing you can do to find laughter within yourself. I have mastered this art and can laugh anytime, anywhere. I have liberated my laughter from all reasons and conditions.

As the laughter movement gained momentum across the world, I found myself spreading the message of laughter and helping people laugh more than ever. There were times when I would travel for over six months in a year, which was very stressful and made me miss my personal laughter moments. Madhuri and I practiced the exercises together, but eventually I decided to do them on my own as she found it difficult to keep up with my erratic hours.

I experimented with laughing alone by trying different positions like sitting, standing and even lying down. I found it easier to laugh with every passing session. Highly motivated, I started laughing alone for twenty to thirty minutes every day with some breaks for deep breathing.

While conducting seminars and training programs in the West, I started teaching the groups how to laugh by themselves. It worked well and soon became popular. Since laughter clubs meet once a week, or every two weeks, in the Western countries, I encouraged my students to laugh alone every day. Many laughter leaders and teachers tried laughing in the bathroom or in front of a mirror with positive results. People loved this new technique, which helped them release stress and maintain good health.

This confirms that laughter yoga not only heals when practiced in a group but also when practiced alone. This exercise regime, which combines laughter and breathing exercises, benefits those who are looking for alternative methods for daily laughter, as well as those suffering from chronic diseases and those unable to move or exercise. Laughing alone is an innovative way of practicing laughter exercises to reap the same health benefits as those enjoyed when one is part of a laughter club.

Factors That Can Help You Laugh Alone

- **Willingness to Laugh:** Laughing on purpose sounds awkward to many people as they feel that it is not genuine laughter. Scientific research has shown that the body generates positive responses even if you have the intention to do something good. Therefore, a willingness to laugh creates a positive mind-set that is necessary to be receptive to the benefits of laughing alone. Injecting exaggerated mannerisms into your laughter will allow suppressed emotions to be released more easily.

- **Self-Dialogue:** Do not criticize the quality of your laughter. Tell yourself that this is not about real or spontaneous laughter, but that it is only an exercise with scientifically proven benefits. Appreciate yourself and pat yourself on the back each time you laugh more and without reason. No other exercise is natural; we do it because we know we will benefit from it. Tell your mind that daily laughter is good for your own health.

- **Forty-Day Formula:** To adopt any new habit, one has to repeat it for least for forty days. This helps develop new circuits in the brain, with the new behavior becoming a part of the subconscious mind. Laughing alone over an extended period of time conditions a joyful state of mind. The brain actually develops new neuronal connections that produce happy neuropeptides and hormones that are triggered by this repetitive act.

Guidelines Before Getting Started

- **Get Over Awkwardness:** Initially you may feel awkward about what others think when you laugh all by yourself. They may think that you are out of your mind. Therefore, before you start laughing, you must tell your family that you are practicing laughter yoga, which is just like any other exercise routine. You can also ask them to join in if they are willing. Even if they are not, at least they will not stop you from doing it once they understand the concept.

- **Every Person Is Different:** Laughter is individualized—there is no right or wrong way to laugh. When laughing alone, you will produce sounds, gestures and postures that you are comfortable with. Create your own exercises and develop new ideas in order to discover what works best for you. Once you start laughing, you will be surprised to see how laughter improves your sense of creativity.

- **What to Wear:** Wear loose and comfortable clothes while doing breathing and laughter exercises. Trousers should be tied below the navel so as not to hinder abdominal movements. Also, avoid tight belts that may restrict belly movement.

- **Duration and Ideal Time:** Ideally, fifteen minutes each should be spent on yogic breathing and laughter sessions with short breaks in between to relax. You can begin with five to ten minutes and gradually increase the duration. Laughing alone should preferably be practiced the first thing every morning since it will put you in a cheerful mood and help you feel good throughout the day. If you do not feel like laughing in the morning, begin with some warm-up and breathing exercises. They will stimulate the body and laughter will follow. This can be done anytime during the day to boost energy levels.

Steps to Laughing Alone Exercises

- **Warm-up Exercise (Ho Ho, Ha Ha)**

Before starting with laughing alone exercises, ensure that you warm up. Exercises like chanting "ho ho" and "ha ha ha" and "very good, very good, yay" are some expressions that you can use. These exercises will be even more fun if you do them alone in front of a mirror. Do them gently in the beginning and gradually increase the intensity until you are comfortable.

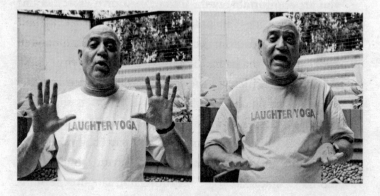

Ideally, this warm-up exercise should be done in a standing position. Say "ho ho" twice as you push your hands away from your chest and say "ha ha" as you push your hands toward the ground (refer to the pictures above). Slowly sway your body from left to right and bend your knees slightly as you say "ho ho" and "ha ha ha" faster. After doing this a couple of times, do some deep-breathing exercises. Raise your arms above your head, inhale and hold your breath for three to five seconds. Then slowly bend at the waist, let your arms dangle and exhale saying "haaaaaaaaa." Continue to laugh after this.

- **Try Different Laughter Sounds**

You can do these while sitting or standing.

a) "Ho Ho" Sounds from the Belly: Put your hand on your belly button. With your mouth open, say "ho ho ho." Feel the movement of your abdominal muscles and let the laughter sounds from your belly stimulate the diaphragm. After a while, increase the speed and burst into laughter while saying "ho ho ho."

b) "Ha Ha" Sounds from the Chest: Place your hand on your heart and say "ha ha ha." Feel the vibrations in your chest. After a while, increase the speed and burst into laughter while saying "ha ha ha."

c) "He He" Sounds from Your Throat: Place your hands on your neck, where your larynx is, and say "he he he." Feel the sound in your throat. Next, burst out laughing and feel the vibrations.

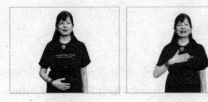

d) Humming into Your Ears: Place both your hands on your ears, close your eyes and mouth and hum. Slowly convert this sound into humming laughter and feel it in your head and deep inside your brain.

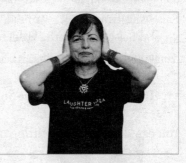

- **Breathe, Hold, Laugh**

This is a very powerful breath-holding technique. Straighten your arms before your chest with the palms facing upward. Inhale through the nose and bring your fists closer to your chest. Hold your breath for three to four seconds and then burst out laughing while exhaling. Repeat thrice (refer to the pictures below).

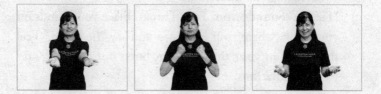

- **Breathing into the Lungs**

a) Breathing into the Upper Lobe: The lungs have three lobes. This exercise will bring more air to the upper lobe. Place your hands between your shoulder blades with the palms facing outward (refer to the pictures below). Take a deep breath, hold for three to four seconds and laugh. Repeat thrice.

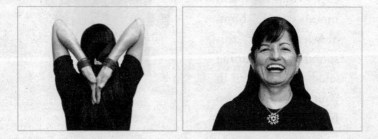

b) Breathing into the Middle Lobe: Join both your palms and stretch them above your head until your arms are straight. This is called the mountain posture in yoga. Take a deep breath, hold it for three to four seconds and laugh. This will oxygenate your middle lobes. Repeat thrice (refer to the pictures below).

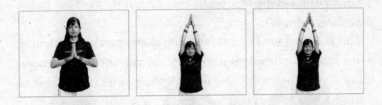

c) Breathing into the Lower Lobe: Hold your hands out like a lion's paws (refer to the pictures below). Take a deep breath, hold it for three to four seconds and then stick your tongue out and laugh from your belly. This will help bring more air into the lower lobe. Repeat thrice.

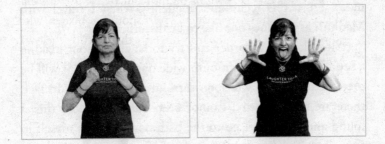

• **Fake It Until You Make It**

Try to fake laughter by saying "ha ha ha," "he he he" and "ho ho ho." Keep doing this till you can laugh genuinely at the sound of your own laughter. Try different ways to fake laughter sounds until you find those that amuse you. Stick to them and practice them often. Initially, simulated laughter may seem awkward, but with repeated practice your body will become conditioned and allow real laughter to follow the moment you start faking it.

- **Gentle Laughter**

This is one of my favorite laughing alone exercises. Laughing out loud on purpose is difficult to sustain for many people. But if you laugh softly and keep giggling, you can continue to laugh for as long as you want and let it sound natural.

- **Silent Laughter**

This is the most useful exercise that anyone can do without disturbing other people. When you know that you have to laugh without making a sound, you end up laughing even more. I use this technique frequently when I travel with Madhuri as she does not like to be disturbed.

Sit quietly in a corner and try to laugh without making a sound, but keep your mouth wide open. Though it will be pretense initially, it will soon turn into real laughter. In fact, there are times when I cannot keep quiet. To avoid this, I found another way. I go to the bathroom, look at myself in the mirror and start laughing silently.

- **Voice Reinforcement Technique**

Have you ever noticed that when you are not in a good mood, you sound low? In contrast, when you are happy and confident, you sound cheerful. Laughter exercises open up your voice, which resets your emotional state through a process called biofeedback. The freedom and expression of one's voice affects the flow of emotions in the mind. Thus, the pitch and tone of your laughter can change your state of mind, even if it is practiced as an exercise. As there is a two-way link between the body and mind, freeing your voice with the sound of laughter can bring about a change in your emotional state.

The two most important laughing alone exercises where you can use this voice reinforcement technique are the one-yard laughter and the aloha laughter. Basically, before laughing we use prolonged vowel sounds like "ayyyy" or "oooooo."

a) Aloha Laughter: This is derived from the traditional Hawaiian greeting and is very stimulating. It allows for increased circulation as the body movements involved in it facilitate the supply of blood to the brain.

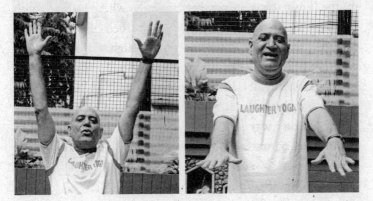

Ideally, it should be performed in the morning, immediately after waking up and preferably on the bed. Sit with your knees bent and place a pillow or two in front of you. With both your arms raised over your head and your chin held up, say a prolonged "aloooooh." End it with a loud "haaa" as you lower your body toward the bed, bending toward the pillows, laughing heartily. Continue laughing for as long you enjoy it (refer to the pictures on the previous page).

Aloha laughter can also be performed while standing. Raise your arms over your head and keeping your chin up say "alooooh." End the exercise by saying "haaaa." Finally, lower your arms and continue laughing.

• Holding Your Knees Laughter

This exercise facilitates the upward movement of the diaphragm by pressing the abdominal muscles. It also helps to increase blood flow to the brain thus improving circulation. It involves pulling the knees toward your chest and releasing them as you exhale and inhale. Lie down on your back, hold your knees together with both your hands and bring them closer to your chest. While doing this, push your 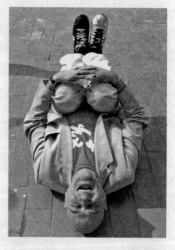 chin upward and keep your mouth a little open to exhale. This helps to straighten the respiratory tract and allows air to flow freely through it. In the next step, release your knees and take deep breaths.

> **Robert Rivest, United States:** I have become more playful, joyful, generous, friendly, peaceful and relaxed since I started doing laughter yoga. I am able to spend more quality time with my family and friends. What I love about my daily laughter practice is that not only does it make me feel calm and peaceful, but it also lets me change my mood within minutes. Physically, too, I feel healthier. I fall sick less often, can exercise more and breathe easier than ever before.
>
> In my early thirties, I suffered from several trauma-induced and stress-related illnesses including post-traumatic stress disorder (PTSD), depression and allergies. Laughter yoga became a major part of my healing process and helped to reduce many of the symptoms. Socially, I have opened up as I am a better listener now—more understanding and compassionate. Professionally, I have benefited tremendously as a performer and speaker. Laughter yoga has given me great control over my breathing and voice quality. It has also let me be of greater service to others.

Integrating Laughter Exercises with Everyday Situations

Laughing alone is a great way to release stress and negative thoughts, to dissipate anger and focus on meditative activities.

Additionally, it aids in boosting self-confidence by reducing shyness. It also helps in dealing with trivial irritants of daily life such as broken vending machines, traffic jams, rude teenagers and long queues in the supermarket. Learning to laugh alone can help you face these "free-floating anxieties" positively.

Laughing alone also lets you communicate effectively by creating a safe environment for others to comfortably connect with you, thus allowing you to enjoy positive relationships in your professional, personal and social life.

- **Laugh Your Way Through Household Chores:** Laugh while doing repetitive household chores such as washing the dishes, mopping the floor, hanging clothes and cleaning windows. You don't need to laugh loudly, even a gentle giggle will help change your perspective toward mundane chores and make them seem less daunting.
- **Laughing in the Bathroom:** Your bathroom can become a safe haven for you to laugh alone. You can be as funny as you want to be without the fear of anyone watching. Laughing while taking a shower will program the body accordingly. The moment you turn on the tap, you will start laughing. This is the benefit of repeating an activity over and over again and combining physical behavior with it.
- **Walking and Laughing:** Gentle laughter can easily be combined with walking and is an additional workout to stimulate blood circulation. If you are worried about

other people watching you laugh as you walk, find some private area and try to let out a few minutes of hearty laughter. I do this regularly while walking. People around me don't mind any more as they all know who I am!

- **Laughing in the Car:** Laughing alone exercises can be used most effectively during trying times on the road. Instead of losing patience, laugh away those situations to release the anger. The "ho ho" and "ha ha ha" exercise works well without sound, but it depends on your level of comfort, as you might become aware of other people watching you laugh. Instead of cursing the driver who cut you off, laugh. He will be shocked and you will feel much better, not to mention that your heart will also thank you.

- **Laugh at Yourself (Ha Ha Mantra):** Laughing at yourself does not degrade you. It is a gentle reminder that we must take ourselves lightly to keep our spirits high. Instead of laughing, say "haaaaa, haaaa, haaaa," dragging out each "ha" a few times. It will make you feel much better as it changes the negative perspective of the situation. I always use this mantra when I mess up or drop food on my shirt or when something falls from my hands.

- **Ha Ha Mantra for Free-floating Hostilities:** These are infuriating situations in daily life that can irritate and cause stress. Combat these with the "ha ha" mantra. Each time you find yourself heading toward a really bad mood, remember to slowly say "haaaaa, haaaaa, haaaa." It can work wonders!

Veronique, Switzerland: Laughing every day in the bathroom has become a routine. It's like taking a shower or brushing my teeth. I feel my brain is more aware of everything around me and my concentration is better. I feel more efficient at my workplace and find myself smiling at everyone and every situation.

Laughter yoga has taught me to be more playful and helped me connect with my true essence, the one I had when I was a teenager. Then life turned me another way: marriage, children, friends, family, social standing and so many other good reasons to become someone else. Laughter yoga brought freedom to me. I'm free to be myself once again with an ability to express emotions better. I can immediately connect with people. I place less boundaries on myself and easily connect with children as laughter helps to cultivate childlike playfulness. Life is easier now.

Physically, laughter yoga has taught me to do deep breathing from the belly, which has helped me improve my health. I can now run for much longer than before and my abdominal muscles are stronger too. Mentally, laughter has increased my confidence levels. As a professional singer, I would always be nervous before going on stage, but laughter and deep-breathing exercises have helped me become less anxious. Laughter has become my first reflex when I am confronted with difficult situations. It allows me to stand back and find solutions.

12

How to Laugh Without Laughing: In Your Mind

"Against the assault of laughter, nothing can stand."

—Mark Twain

It is easy to laugh when everything is fine, but there may be situations when it becomes very difficult to do so. For example, how do you laugh when you are sick, admitted to a hospital, recuperating after surgery or going through emotional stress?

Here is the answer: yes, it is hard to laugh in tough situations, but there is no need to laugh out loud or do laughter exercises. Laughter can be programmed into your body and mind. Simply imagining that you are laughing can trigger the release of happy chemicals, which will have the same effect. Several years ago, when I underwent surgery for a herniated disk, my recovery was quick as I kept laughing in my mind. This technique is called Mind Sound Resonance Technique (MSRT). I learned it at the Swami Vivekananda Yoga Anusandhana Samasthana

(S-VYASA) in Bengaluru. It allows you to program your mind when you are healthy so that you cope better with sickness.

What Is MSRT?

As part of this technique you need to produce a particular sound, then close your eyes and reproduce it in your mind, breathing normally all the while. Please note that when you actually produce the sound, you need to exhale for as long as you do so. However, when you produce the sound in the mind, you can do it irrespective of whether you are inhaling or exhaling. It is not the production of the sound in the mind that is important; it is feeling the resonance of that sound in your body that is more important. You can try this with any musical note, mantra or even vowel sounds such as "aa, eeee, ooooo." Take a deep breath and produce this sound with your eyes closed to feel it within your body. Now do the same, but in your mind, while breathing normally. Try to feel the resonance in your body. It might take a few weeks of practice before you can train your mind and body.

Programming with Laughter

Laughter sounds can be programmed like any other sound. In fact, it is better if laughter sounds follow a particular rhythm. For example, in the one-yard laughter we say "aay" thrice and then burst out laughing saying "ha ha ha." After you finish laughing, try the same in your mind with your eyes closed. You can also try doing this two to three times. Other laughter exercises that have rhythmic properties are the milkshake and aloha laughter. When doing it in your mind, you will be able to feel the vibrations in your body. Another thing I noticed while laughing in my mind was that I could retain a smile as a result.

Throughout our lives, we are conditioned in both positive and negative ways. We develop several belief systems and superstitions that alter our physiology and bio-chemistry.

Here Are a Few Examples

In India, there is a popular superstition that anything important done on a Saturday or a Tuesday is bound to go wrong. Even if something goes wrong coincidentally, your mind accepts it as something that was expected.

In another example, if your boss is short-tempered, most people may naturally become fearful of him/her. Under such circumstances, if you are asked to meet him/her, your body will produce stress chemicals without being aware of the reason why you have been called. Over a period of time, and with more repetitions of similar behavior, your mind is programmed in a way that leads you to be fearful of your boss to an extent that even seeing his/her car can get your body to respond negatively. In fact, seeing any car that is similar to your boss's will cause your body to react.

Most of the conditioning in our life is negative and happens by default. But we can program our body and mind. What we need to do is to create a positive situation. Doing

laughter exercises is a positive experience, and regular
practitioners of laughter yoga become conditioned to being
joyful. Clapping in rhythm, chanting "ho ho" and "ha ha ha"
in unison, and positive affirmations like "very good, very
good, yay" are a few examples of expressions of joy that can be
practiced repeatedly.

13

Join or Create a Social Laughter Club

"Laughter clubs are like kindergarten for grown-ups."

Quality of life does not depend on how much money, power and success you have. Rather, it depends on our relationships with the people around us. In times of both success and failure, we need people to share our joy and sorrow. It is often seen that the family is unable to provide the happiness and security that a good friend can. This establishes the fact that the best relationships are mostly shared with friends who are always around to provide unconditional love and support.

Loneliness is the biggest social disorder today. No one has time for anybody else; people are busy with work and other commitments that keep them occupied. The younger generation hardly relates to their parents as mobile technology and social media leaves them with no time. Social laughter clubs are platforms that provide an opportunity to remedy this growing malady of living in a virtual world. It provides a platform for people to meet and develop a social circle. Laughter attracts like-minded people and is an excellent tool to bring them together like an extended family.

Laughter yoga practitioners laugh together daily or weekly. The healing effects are different for each person according to their physical, mental and emotional needs. Besides experiencing the therapeutic power of laughter, people also experience a profound change in their mental condition as it helps them counter depression, anxiety and stress. Members have reported moving from debilitating fear and anxiety to a more positive state of mind. Many others who harbored feelings of bitterness, hatred and other long-term emotional problems found that all their pent-up feelings were released through the cathartic effects of laughter, leaving them joyful and free.

People suffering from life-threatening diseases such as cancer also find laughter to be a refuge to deal with the trauma and pain. Even students with emotional problems, which leave them incapable of learning, have reported that laughter helped them continue their education and do well.

What Is a Laughter Club?

Laughter clubs are the heart and soul of the laughter yoga movement. They are a worldwide network of social clubs run by volunteers. People get together in groups in public places or indoor venues and practice laughter exercises, along with breathing and stretching exercises, to reap enormous health benefits. These clubs are free and connect people from different cultures and countries, no matter what language they speak.

Developing Close-Knit Communities

With the spread of laughter clubs worldwide, the members experience a sense of affiliation and belonging to the group. In fact, these clubs are fast becoming close-knit communities. The members not only care for others' happiness but also share their sorrows, thus reinforcing a feeling of belonging to a caring community. This is the kind of "laughing family" that the world needs. A laughter club, in many ways, provides a protective shell that safeguards our emotional well-being. It has brought a lot of people together and created the awareness that one is not alone.

Many members with chronic pain, migraines, headaches and asthma have found the attacks to become less frequent, and in some cases, to disappear completely. Symptoms of high blood pressure, severe spinal, neck or shoulder problems and even diabetes have improved eventually.

Examples to Prove the Strong Bonding Power of These Clubs

A laughter club member from Mumbai was devastated when his uninsured shop was burned down. He was ruined; the result of twenty-five years of hard work was down the drain. He was left in debt and with no means to support his family. Members of his laughter club came together to raise money and rebuild his shop and provide for new stock.

In another case, an elderly member of a laughter club was left shattered when her husband of more than forty years passed away. She had got married early in life and had never worked outside her home. She went into depression, refused food and did not leave her bed. Her fellow laughter club members arranged for medical care and took turns staying with her throughout the day, bringing her treats and cajoling her to eat. But most importantly, they were there for her. After three months, she recovered. Convinced that her life would have ended without a laughter club, she started a new club at a school nearby where she conducts daily sessions for students.

Another example is that of a senior member of a laughter club in Mumbai who fell sick and was admitted to a hospital. He burst into tears of joy when he found his room at the hospital flooded with flowers from the members of the laughter club, that too when none of his relatives turned up to visit him.

In another incident, Mr. Mingo, a laughter leader from Taiwan, met with an unfortunate road accident after finishing a laughter session on May 3, 2010, a day after World Laughter Day. His fellow laughter club members visited him regularly in the hospital and gave him the love and energy required to recover quickly.

Spiritual Benefits of Laughter Clubs

In addition to providing a positive and secure emotional environment, laughter clubs also promote personal happiness in many ways. Members of these clubs are able to spread positivity and happiness through the mechanism of emotional contagion. This is not limited to just friends, family and co-workers but also includes social contacts and people who sit next to us in a bus or a restaurant.

Their caring, empathetic manner touches all those they interact with, thus letting the benefits continue. Laughter allows emotional problems and selfish interests to disappear and fills the heart with joy.

This inner spirit of laughter becomes apparent to some people as they develop a state of emotional fluidity where worries and goals that drive their lives become less important to them. These people become aware that true happiness comes from giving unconditional love, sharing and working to make the world a better place not only for themselves but for everyone.

Finding a Laughter Club

In India, most public parks hold laughter club sessions in the morning. If you find a group of people laughing, do not hesitate to join them—it's free. To find clubs in other countries, log on to www.laughteryoga.org.

How to Start a Laughter Club

In India, most laughter clubs function on a daily basis with the members meeting at public parks. If you want to start a laughter club, find a place in your locality where people can assemble. It can be a public park, an open ground or a beach. The advantage of selecting such a place is that you can combine laughter yoga sessions with your morning walk.

The chosen venue should not be in the vicinity of residential complexes. In areas where weather conditions are not favorable throughout the year, it is not possible to conduct laughter sessions regularly. Under such circumstances, these sessions can be held during yoga classes at health clubs or at aerobic centers where laughter can be a value addition to the ongoing activities.

Laughter Yoga in Western Countries

The concept of laughter clubs is slightly different in the West, where club members like to meet for two hours every weekend or fortnightly. They laugh together for thirty minutes along with breathing and stretching exercises, followed by laughter meditation for thirty minutes. After that, they participate in activities, games, brainstorming on psychological and philosophical aspects of laughter and dancing. The frequency of such laughter meetings can be decided based on the convenience of the group.

14

Laugh Online Every Day with Skype Laughter Clubs

"An optimist laughs to forget, a pessimist forgets to laugh."

—Tom Nansbury

What Are Skype Laughter Clubs?

With laughter yoga becoming more and more popular, the number of people looking to practice it is also increasing. Thanks to technology, there are new ways of doing so. Among these are Skype laughter clubs, which are coming up almost every hour according to different time zones. These clubs are an online community of laughter lovers who connect and practice laughter yoga for fifteen to twenty minutes each day.

The laughter sessions involve free-flowing laughter rather than guided exercises and are conducted by a team of passionate laughter enthusiasts who volunteer on a rotational basis. These leaders are usually, but not always, laughter yoga teachers.

Remember: you will be able to enjoy maximum benefits if you laugh every day.

How to Join a Free Skype Laughter Club?

Skype laughter clubs are free of charge and easy to join. All you need is a computer with the Skype app installed—you can download it on www.skype.com—a good Internet connection and a headset, microphone or speakers.

- Add "laughterclub" to your Skype contacts. Please wait for your request to be accepted.
- Choose a convenient time according to your time zone. You will find a list of laughter sessions on our website.
- Before starting a session, the coordinator of the Skype laughter club will send out a message inviting all online contacts to join. If you wish to be a part of the session, please send a message saying "I am in. Ho ho, ha ha ha. Please call." You may also send a smiley emoticon. You will get a call at the scheduled time.

Maria Manninen, Finland: For a while, my life was so tough that I spent a lot of time crying alone at home. I decided to join a Skype laughter club and anxiously waited for the first session. In just a couple of weeks, my life started to fill up with joy and laughter. I found myself smiling and laughing throughout the day. When something was funny, I would laugh out loud, which I hardly did before. After a Skype laughter session, I feel so much happier. In fact, sometimes I laugh so much that I have to explain to people that I'm a laughter yoga practitioner!

The Experience of Skype Laughter Clubs

A Skype laughter club conducts sessions over a conference call where members laugh for no reason and focus on laughter as an exercise. You can laugh gently, hear others laughing and wait for your laughter to become spontaneous. Even if it does not, just keep laughing. Of course you can take breaks and take deep breaths while you hear the others laugh.

Although these clubs are consistent with the laughter yoga expectation of "laughing and not talking," there exists a culture of instant messaging throughout the duration of the Skype call. This allows the group members to get to know each other.

I feel that following and/or engaging in a conversation on the side takes me out of the laughter zone. If you are like me and prefer to listen to laughter and enter a state of free-flowing laughter, simply minimize the chat section. You can always chat at the end when people start to say good-bye.

Usually, we do not encourage people to opt for a video chat as it affects the quality of transmission. However, if there are less than ten people left at the end of a session, you can participate in a video chat and say hello to each other. If your call drops during the session, you can call again and join the group, or send a chat message saying "please call."

Make sure that there is no disturbance in the background. Let the laughter be pure. You can, nevertheless, use funny props like hats, talk gibberish or make animal sounds.

> **Brigitte Kottwitz, Germany:** A big change happened to me a year and a half ago when I started participating in Skype laughter sessions every day. Today, one hour of laughter gives me the energy and strength to go to work with pleasure. It helps me handle daily pressures with ease. I have also connected with other laughter friends who play an important role in the lives of people like me who don't have families. I receive encouragement and support during times of illness and difficult decisions. Everyone in the group is positive toward the others.

Facilitator's Guidelines:

- **Dos**

a) Be regular and punctual. It helps to be online a few minutes before the session to organize the group and answer the queries of newcomers. Ensure the Internet connection is proper and there is no disturbance in the background. Start with gentle gradient laughter and be alert to the messages popping up.

b) Welcome the participants warmly and thank everybody at the end for joining the session.

c) You can advertise the session on the Facebook page "Skype laughterclub."

d) Remind the participants to take a few deep breaths during the session.

e) Be friendly and caring toward the participants and help the newcomers.

f) Put your heart and soul into each session.

g) Have an alternate Internet connection as standby, if possible.

h) Inform the "Skype laughterclub leaders" group in advance if you won't be able to conduct a session so that someone else can substitute for you.

• **Don'ts**

a) Please don't send group invitations. It can annoy members who do not wish to participate.

b) Do not add people without their consent.

c) Don't worry if there are few people in a session.

d) Don't mimic participants or make fun of them.

e) There should be no talking gibberish or singing at the beginning of a session.

f) Don't end the session abruptly.

Anu Saari, Finland: A Skype laughter club gives me the chance to laugh every day as part of a group. A laughter session helps when you have had a tough day after which laughing alone is hard, or when you find all the excuses not to do so. It makes it easier to get yourself to laugh and gives gray lazy mornings an energy boost. I have also made great friends around the world—shared laughter really warms the heart!

15

Four Strategies to Bring More Laughter into Your Life

"He who laughs, lasts!"

—Mary Pettibone Poole

The core philosophy of laughter yoga is not to seek happiness but to cultivate joy. Happiness is a concept that depends on a variety of things, all of which, for the most part, are fleeting. Absolutely happy people are rare. Conversely, joy can be triggered by the simplest of physical activities such as singing, dancing, playing or laughing. All of these are an integral part of laughter yoga and are called the four elements of joy.

Children are born with these basic elements intact. Unfortunately, as we grow older, inhibitions and self-consciousness limit participation in joyful activities. Laughter yoga has the ability to revive these elements and make it easier for people to participate in fun activities.

Singing

Singing helps express emotions. Music has a major impact on life and affects both behavior and mind-set. Soothing strains of music are a panacea for a tired soul and body, capable of releasing stress and changing a negative state of mind. Also, it can act as a catharsis for pent-up feelings. Laughter yoga uses singing and music routinely to bring an inner sense of joy, as well as to help people connect and bond while overcoming self-consciousness and reticence.

Medical studies have shown that singing can lower heart rate and blood pressure, relieve asthma, improve lung capacity, reduce stress and pain, and enhance relaxation. Extensive studies focusing on the elderly have found that singing makes breathing easier, improves posture and decreases the number of visits to a doctor. Singing also benefits those who suffer from dementia, Alzheimer's disease or memory loss by tapping into that area of the brain where long-forgotten words are stored. There have been instances of patients who were unable to string two meaningful words together recalling words to an entire song. Singing in a group, plus the realization that they can recall things, nearly always elevates their mood.

As a child growing up in a small village in India, I remember listening to and watching my mother as she went about her daily chores with a song on her lips. From the time she woke up at 4 a.m. to take care of her eight children and five farm workers, she sang. I now understand that she used singing as a form of meditation that allowed her to manage what would otherwise have been a difficult and stressful life. In India, music is a major part of culture. Not only do Indians constantly come together to sing, but they also chant together. A classic example of this is farmers who sing together while working in the fields.

Getting Over Roadblocks

Most people love to sing but think that they are not good singers. They feel that singing is a special talent. But this is not true. You don't have to be a professional singer to sing. For instance, when we sing national anthems and devotional songs, we don't bother with the melody. This shows that it is very easy to sing in a group. It is when we sing individually that we become self-conscious and feel that we will judged for our voice.

In laughter yoga, singing in a group is a regular practice. Most people get used to singing even if they have never sung in their whole life.

Practical Suggestions to Cultivate Singing Habits

- **Group Singing:** Try to be enthusiastic whenever you get an opportunity to sing in a group, irrespective of whether it is a religious, cultural or social occasion.
- **Sing-along:** For beginners, it is easy to sing along with the radio or any recorded music. Keep the music on while working at home and sing along.
- **Bathroom Singing:** In the beginning, take the radio with you into the shower and slowly start singing on your own. Nobody will judge you when you are in the bathroom.
- **Sing with Children:** You can learn a lot from children. Try to sing nursery rhymes and jingles with them to become less self-conscious.
- **Karaoke:** Try karaoke. You don't even have to buy the equipment, all you need is YouTube. Just play and sing along.

- **Try Humming:** Listen to your favorite songs and try to hum along. Since there are no words involved in humming, you will feel more confident.
- **Whistling:** Try to whistle to a few lines of your favorite song if you know how to do it.
- **Tongue Twisters:** Learn some tongue twisters and try to get them right with your family and friends.
- **Drumming on Tabletops:** Along with singing, try drumming on tabletops, utensils, empty bottles, etc. and try to create an orchestra. Enjoy these music sessions with your family and friends.
- **Organize Horrible Singing Contests:** Just to have fun, ask people to sing in the most horrible manner they can. This will definitely make everyone laugh.
- **Sing Gibberish:** Speak gibberish and try to create a melody out of it.

Vowel Sound Meditation

Do this for five to ten minutes. In India, chanting mantras is a popular way of meditation as it has a calming effect on the mind and body. If you study these mantras, you will observe that they use vowel sounds quite often. In laughter yoga, we have discovered a non-religious way of chanting mantras, which we call vowel sound meditation.

How to Go About It?

Sit in a comfortable position on the floor or on a chair. Close your eyes and feel your body relax from head to toe.

- Take a deep breath and start chanting the first vowel "a" (phonetically, it will sound like the "a" in "say" and "day"). Keep chanting until you run out of breath. Try to feel the sound resonate in your body. Repeat this five times.
- Chant the second vowel "e" and move on to "i," "o" and "u." Do this five times.
- Try humming and feel the resonance in your body.
- The basic rule is to inhale as deeply as you can. Fill up your lungs with a lot of air and release it by singing slowly until you run out of breath. This allows you to slow down your breathing rate, which relaxes your body and mind. Normally, we breathe fifteen to seventeen times per minute, but chanting these vowel sounds will bring it down to just six to eight times per minute.

Dancing

If singing is good for you, dancing is even better. In addition to all the benefits of singing, dancing goes several steps further. It increases flexibility, improves range of motion, builds muscle and keeps joints lubricated, thus keeping arthritis at bay. It improves balance, burns calories and is a great aerobic exercise. Additionally, it is a social activity that increases self-esteem and self-confidence, facilitating a feeling of well-being.

Perhaps most impressive is the study published in the *New England Journal of Medicine* which found that dancing can reduce the risk of Alzheimer's disease and other forms of dementia in the elderly. According to the study, those over the age of seventy-five who engaged in reading, dancing and playing musical instruments and board games at least once a week had a 7 percent lower risk of dementia compared to those who did not. However, those who participated in these activities at least eleven days a month had a 63 percent lower risk. Interestingly, dancing was the only physical activity out of the eleven the study considered that was associated with a lower risk of dementia. I guess it's time to put your dancing shoes on![1]

Dancing is an integral part of Indian culture. Any celebration, be it a wedding, festival or social get-together, is not complete without dancing. With so much diversity in culture, there is always some festival every month that provides ample opportunity to dance.

Practical Ideas to Help You Dance More

- **Dance As If There Are No Steps:** Most people feel that they must learn how to dance before they can do so. This is true for professional dancers and performers, but not for casual dancing. Just move the way you want to, as if nobody is watching. Consider dancing to be an expression of your feelings and emotions and move freely. Develop your own style and dance for yourself, not for others.
- **Consider Dancing to Be an Aerobic Exercise:** When you dance as part of a workout, it becomes easier because you are not worried about the steps. It is like dancing for health rather than showing off your talent. Also, people

will not expect you to be a great dancer, which can take the pressure off your mind.

- **Join Dancing Classes:** If you have never danced before, it's a good idea to join dancing classes and learn different styles. This will build confidence and allow you to participate in celebrations.
- **Be the First to Dance:** At social gatherings, people always wait for the others to get up and dance. Be the first to jump onto the dance floor and motivate the others too.
- **Collection of Dance Music:** Keep collecting good music with stimulating beats that motivate you to dance. Also, when you invite people over for any occasion, encourage them to dance.

Playing

Several years ago, I was interviewed by a journalist in New York. At the end, he challenged me with a question: "Dr. Kataria, can you, in just one sentence, say something about laughter and what you have learned in so many years of laughter yoga experience?"

I replied spontaneously. "Why one sentence? I'll tell you in one word. The answer is PLAY."

"Play" is the essence of laughter; its very source of laughter. Who are the best laughers in the world? It is children.

When do children laugh the most? It is when they are playing. The entire concept of laughter yoga is based on cultivating childlike playfulness. But sadly, as we grow older we begin to take life more and more seriously. This is one of the reasons why we lose our ability to laugh.

Playful people have the remarkable ability to adapt to any situation. They have a lot of physical energy and can work for hours together without getting tired. They can also concentrate better and are always bubbling with enthusiasm. At the same time, they have the ability to rest and recharge their bodies and minds quickly. They are also emotionally more intelligent.

Creativity: A Dynamic Energy

Creativity is not born in a vacuum. It is a dynamic energy that is an outcome of movement and play. In other words, creativity can be defined as playing with ideas in your mind. As the body and mind are connected, your mind moves better if you are physically active. Tony Buzan, a brain expert from the UK, says that children are 72 percent creative, while adults are only 22 percent creative. This is because children are physically more active.

Practical Suggestions to Cultivate Playfulness

- **Don't Wait for External Events to Be Joyful:** Joy can be yours right away. It resides within you. It simply needs a reason to spring forth. Therefore, learn to play. It is not a waste of time; rather it is a necessary component of healthy living.
- **Find a Hobby:** Try to cultivate an activity that involves body movement. Choose an activity that will sharpen a skill, something that will enable you to express

your creativity or give you the freedom to blow off steam.

- **Be with Children:** The more you play with children, the more you will be inspired to encourage your inner child. Children can teach you how to keep your grown-up mind aside and have fun. You don't have to analyze what is funny and what is not. When you are with children, everything sounds funny. You cannot engage with children without playing with them.

- **Engage in Regular Sports Activity:** Engaging in non-competitive sporting activities is conducive to good health and keeps your spirits up.

- **Learn Some Fun Games:** Always be on the lookout for new games for when you invite people over. It is a joyful experience that can make you laugh. You can find plenty of ideas on the Internet.

- **Some More Ideas:** Build sand castles, blow bubbles, imitate a clown, climb a tree if possible, doodle or draw cartoons, fly a kite, speak gibberish, have a pillow fight, have an outdoor water fight, have theme days, jump into mud puddles, listen to happy music, make funny faces and sounds, play charades, buy silly props at a costume shop, engage in physical play such as jump rope or hopscotch, recall your most embarrassing moment, end each sentence with "ha," try juggling, try lip-syncing with the sound turned off on your TV and wear funny costumes and hats.

Laughing

There is no right or wrong way to laugh. The important thing is to do it. Explore all possible ways that can bring more laughter into your life. Apart from laughter exercises, you must also look for opportunities that can make you laugh. Keep in mind that you don't laugh at somebody else's expense.

Practical Ideas on How to Find Laughter in Everyday Situations

If you want to laugh more, you have to be mindful of everyday situations that can help you find more laughter in daily life. Here are some ideas:

- **Surround Yourself with Happy People:** It is a scientifically proven fact that your mood and state of mind are affected by the emotions of others. Since happiness is infectious, align yourself with someone who makes you laugh a lot and try to spend more time with that person. If you sense you are inhibiting the laughter of those others around you, apologize and let them know when you are ready to laugh again. Once you open the door to laughter, miracles will happen.
- **Find Friends Who Make You Laugh:** All of us have friends who can make us laugh a lot. Try to identify them and make a commitment to be with them as much as possible. Friendship is the best relationship

one can have. Your friends will be there when you need to share your joy and sorrow. Therefore, invest your time in finding good friends and nurture them.

- **Laugh with Your Family, Laugh at Work:** Laugh at home, laugh with your spouse and children, laugh alone, laugh with your co-workers and laugh with strangers. Turn that frown upside down. Laughter increases endorphin and serotonin levels while decreasing stress hormones. One of my students, who was known to be quite serious before she became a laughter yoga teacher, often tells the story of how she engages her employees in laughter. This transformed her workplace and the attitude of her employees. Not only did she laugh with everyone, she also began and ended every meeting with laughter.

- **Seek Out Humor-Related Entertainment:** Be a laughter magnet. Seek out a humorous TV show, movie or book, listen to a silly song, play a funny game, go to a comedy club, look at silly pictures or visit a funny website. Make laughing a priority. Find humor in everyday situations— in people's behavior and the ridiculousness of certain situations—and laugh out loud.

- **Engage in Fun Activities:** Choose new activities that highlight your playfulness and then laugh at yourself. Exaggerate simple mistakes, be spontaneous—the element of surprise can be hilarious. Physical activity positively affects your mood and can be a source of laughter. If physically able, try fun activities such as dancing, skating or hula-hooping. Theme or costume parties can also be fun. Why not throw one for absolutely no reason? They are always guaranteed to induce plenty of laughter. Gather your friends and family for playing games, sharing funny stories.

- **Act Silly:** One of the reasons people can't laugh is because they are shy and self-conscious around others. It is difficult for them to come out of their comfort zone and try something silly. I suggest you try being silly in a subtle way. For example, you can wear mismatched socks, a red clown nose or attend a costume party. Once you are comfortable, you can try out more acts of silliness in public. I wear black-and-white shoes while traveling around the world and it makes hundreds of people laugh.

- **Learn from Your Pets:** If you want to learn something about playfulness and unconditional love, think of adopting a pet. My dog, Daisy, has helped me a lot when it comes to relaxing and playing. I make the whole world laugh and she makes me laugh. When I run out of ideas while writing, I take a break to play with Daisy. This brings back my creativity and allows ideas to flow again. Even if I come home after just half an hour, she greets me as if I have not met her for ages, which is what we call unconditional love.

- **Buy Humor Props:** Humor props are excellent tools that can highlight the importance of laughter and fun. In our trainings, we always have "fun nights" when people wear funny costumes and makeup, and then go for a "silly walk" and interact with strangers. Visit fun shops and buy humor props and silly costumes that can be used for parties and get-togethers. Keep laughter bags, which make a funny sound when pressed, and hats in your car to remind yourself not to get stressed, especially in a traffic jam. You can also practice laughter and inspire others around you to do the same.

- **Funny Caller Tunes on Your Cell Phone:** Nowadays, several caller tunes are available that can not only make you laugh but also lift the spirits of those trying to contact you.

Part IV

BENEFITS OF LAUGHTER YOGA

16

Laughter and Stress: Physiological Opposites

"If laughter cannot solve your problems,
it will definitely dissolve them."

Stress is associated with almost 90 percent of all illnesses and 80 percent of all prescribed drugs sold. Depression, anxiety, asthma, alcohol and drug addictions, heart disease, diabetes, hypertension and cancer are just some of the major stress-related illnesses prevalent today. It is recognized as the world's biggest killer and costs organizations billions of dollars each year in medical costs, medical leave and loss of performance. Despite the seriousness of it all, we still need some amount of stress or pressure to motivate us to perform well and to help us get away from unpleasant situations. But, if stress is intense and prolonged, it increases the risk of health problems that can be life-threatening at times. To escape stress, people turn to alcohol, smoking and drugs. Though there are many way to reduce and manage stress, laughter is the quickest of them all.

Stress Is Hardwired

In the prehistoric age, stress would occur once in a while and go away as the situation would dissipate. But stress in the modern times is constant because most pressurizing situations are imaginary, not real. This leads to stress becoming hardwired, which triggers sustained release of chemicals that can have exceedingly harmful physiological and psychological effects.

Whenever our mind perceives threat, a part of our brain called the hypothalamus sends out a message to the pituitary gland to release a neurotransmitter called adrenocorticotropic hormone, which stimulates the adrenal glands. These glands secrete stress hormones that prepare our body for "fight or flight" response by increasing the heart rate, elevating blood pressure and blood sugar levels to boost energy supplies. This helps us overcome any critical situation. Moreover, it shuts down a number of important body systems not required for fight or flight action, which include the immune, circulatory, digestive and sexual systems.

Stress Cocktail

The human body responds to stress with a massive release of hormones from the adrenal medulla (epinephrine and norepinephrine) and the adrenal cortex (cortisol) into the bloodstream, which speed up the heart rate, breathing rate, blood pressure and metabolism. The blood vessels open wider to let more blood flow to the large muscle groups, putting them on alert. The pupils dilate to improve vision, the liver releases stored glucose to increase energy and sweat is produced to cool the body. This is known as stress response. It enhances a person's ability to perform well under pressure. However, this response can cause problems when it overreacts or fails to turn off and reset properly. Excess of stress hormones have powerful negative effects on our bodies. Here is how the stress hormones affect our physiology:

- **Cortisol:** This stress hormone leads to impaired cognitive performance, suppressed thyroid function, blood sugar imbalances such as hyperglycaemia, decreased bone density, decrease in muscle tissue, increased blood pressure, lowered immunity, inflammatory responses and memory problems. High cortisol levels also lead to increased abdominal fat, which is associated with a greater number of health problems than fat in other areas of the body. Health problems associated with increased abdominal fat are heart attacks, strokes, development of "bad" cholesterol (LDL) and lower levels of "good" cholesterol (HDL), which in turn leads to other health problems. Repeated increase in cortisol levels leads to depression-like behavior and greater signs of anxiety, especially in males.
- **Catecholamines:** These are immuno-suppressive hormones released when an individual is stressed. They include epinephrine (adrenaline), norepinephrine and dopamine. Catecholamines cause general physiological changes that prepare the body for physical activity (fight or flight response). Some typical effects are increase in heart rate, blood pressure and blood glucose levels.

However, too much of catecholamines harm the body and its immune system. Epinephrine suppresses the immune system and can lead to irregular heartbeats. Norepinephrine increases heart rate and blood pressure and creates a sense of panic and overwhelming fear. It is associated with loss of alertness, poor memory and depression. Moderately high levels of norepinephrine can cause worry, anxiety, increased startle reflex, jumpiness, fear of crowds and small places, impaired concentration, restless sleep and other changes. Physical symptoms include fatigue, muscle tension/cramps, irritability and a sense of being on edge. Almost all anxiety disorders involve norepinephrine elevation. High concentrations of norepinephrine lead to panic attacks. The symptoms include palpitations, a pounding heart or rapid heart rate, sweating and body temperature changes, trembling or shaking, shortness of breath, choking sensation, chest pain and discomfort, nausea or stomach distress, dizziness, light-headedness, fainting, a sense of unreality, fear of losing control or going crazy, fear of dying, numbness and tingling throughout the body and chills and hot flushes.

Symptoms of Stress

A nagging ache at the base of the neck, frequent headaches with tender temples, lethargy and constant fatigue, frequent coughs and colds, stomach knots, nausea and indigestion, irritable bowel or constipation, muscle tension with backache and neck ache, difficulty in sleeping, waking up early, breathlessness, bouts of dizziness, light-headedness, increase/decrease in appetite, increased smoking or drinking, loss of sexual drive, frequent mood swings, feeling of isolation, lack of self-worth, frequent memory lapses, poor decision-making abilities, irritability and aggression, difficulty in concentrating on and allotting priorities and suicidal tendencies are all symptoms of stress.

All of us suffer from some of these symptoms off and on, but if they persist, you need to unwind and laugh more. People try a number of relaxation techniques such as exercise, massage, yoga, meditation, going on holidays, picnics and outings. All these measures are time-consuming and expensive. One needs concentration and the willpower to stick to these pursuits. In fact, most exercise programs are abandoned due to boredom and lack of motivation.

How Laughter Alleviates Stress

Stress and laughter are physiological opposites. You cannot laugh and be stressed at the same time because they activate opposite branches of the autonomic nervous system. Stress activates the sympathetic nervous system, which is the fight or flight response—the system that lets us respond to emergencies. Laughter activates the parasympathetic system, also known as the "rest and digest" system that is responsible for relaxation and rejuvenation.

The predominance of one tends to suppress the other. Laughter quickly reduces the level of stress chemicals and hormones in our body. Significant reductions can occur within minutes and last for days. It switches on and boosts physiological systems that stress switches off, including the circulatory, digestive, sexual and immune systems. Stress, worry, fear and emotional problems stifle learning ability, creativity, teamwork, productivity, efficiency and motivation while laughter strengthens these attributes.

Laughter Cocktail

Laughter triggers the release of a cocktail of chemicals and hormones that are extremely beneficial and crucial to good health. This includes natural killer (NK) cells, endorphins, serotonin, growth hormone, interferon-gamma (IFN) and a host of other beneficial chemicals that are produced every time we laugh heartily for extended periods.

Laughter boosts the immune responses, particularly components related to antiviral and antitumor defense. It diminishes the secretion of cortisol and epinephrine while enhancing immune reactivity. It boosts secretion of the growth hormone, which enhances key immune responses. The physiological effects of a single laughter session can last twenty-four hours, and regular sessions can produce profound and long-lasting changes. It also reduces the symptoms of depression and prevents many diseases and disorders caused by chronic stress.

- **Endorphins:** These are our bodies' natural painkillers. The name means "morphine made by the body." Laughter stimulates production of endorphins, which create a pleasant "high" feeling and also act as an effective painkiller. Beta endorphins produce a sense of well-being, reduce pain, ease emotional distress, increase self-esteem and even create a sense of euphoria.

- **Serotonin:** This makes you feel mellow, relaxed, hopeful and optimistic. You have a sense of being at peace with life. You are creative, thoughtful and focused. You also have better control over impulses, which enables you to say "no" more easily.

- **Growth Hormone:** This increases calcium retention and strengthens and increases the mineralization of bones. It increases muscle mass and protein synthesis and growth of different organ systems, resulting in a "positive nitrogen balance." The hormone stimulates the immune system and improves liver and digestive functions besides reducing body fat. A recent medical study has shown that growth hormone levels increased by 87 percent after laughter.

- **NK cells:** These are best known for their capacity to kill tumor cells before they become established cancers. They are also important in controlling microbial infections and viral attacks. NK cells are the first line of defense against cancer and infectious diseases. They constitute a major component of the immune system and defend the body against viruses and other pathogens. Psychoneuroimmunology studies have concluded that laughter dramatically and immediately increases the number of NK cells.

- **IFN:** This activates T cells, B cells, immunoglobulins and NK cells. It helps to fight viruses and regulate cell growth. It fights tumorous cells, including cancer. Blood samples taken before, during and after laughter exercises have shown a significant increase in IFN levels lasting into the following day.

Dominique Toulet, New Caledonia: I work as a conference interpreter from English to French. It is a profession recognized for being stressful. I sometimes work with the heads of states and the like, and the work can be a real source of stress, particularly when the stakes are really high. As a laughter yoga teacher, I systematically devote half an hour to breathing (five pranayama exercises) and half an hour to laughter meditation before each conference. I find it boosts my confidence more than anything else. I go to work happy, calm and ready to deliver to the best of my abilities with no fear, stage fright or negative feeling to affect my performance. Laughter is the best mood and confidence enhancer I know of.

Linda Leclerc, Canada: I tell people that laughter helps reduce stress levels and relieve tension. Whenever I feel nervous before meeting a new group or making a presentation, I lock myself in the bathroom and do my "survival routine" exercises: a few deep breaths, two to three minutes of silent laughter, stretching and breathing. Then I do one minute of lion laughter, take a few deep breaths and am ready to go! Every time I do this, it is like a discovery for me. It really works!

17

Laughter Yoga for Wellness

"Laughter is like mental floss.
It clears the cobwebs of our minds."

The demand for laughter yoga has grown exponentially in the last two decades. More and more people want to be involved with it because they are motivated by the health benefits it offers. People want to practice laughter yoga on a daily basis, which is leading to an increase in the number of social laughter clubs around the world. Laughter yoga can also be called instant yoga because people feel the benefits from the very first session and it triggers an improvement in physical, mental and emotional well-being.

The benefits of laughter yoga can be divided into two categories: preventive and therapeutic. It has all the elements of a perfect health-building activity. It is not the concept or the philosophy that attracts people; it is what they get and how it benefits them. In this chapter, we will talk about the preventive benefits of laughter and how it helps to improve quality of life and contributes to personal growth.

Laughter Yoga for Fitness

One of the reasons people fall sick is lack of exercise. Also, most exercise programs become monotonous and boring after a while. People don't feel motivated to continue the exercises, which are a lot of hard work. That is why we call it a workout. It has been found that most treadmill machines are used regularly for two months, after which they are used to hang clothes. One of the great things about laughter yoga is that one can enjoy benefits similar to any other aerobic exercise, that too without sweating it out on the jogging track. Moreover, laughter exercises are a lot of fun for the person practicing it as well as for those who are watching.

Best Cardio Workout

As life becomes more sedentary and stressful, people find it hard to stick to an exercise routine, making laughter yoga an ideal alternative. It can be compared to any other aerobic exercise, except that you don't have to wear fancy shoes or clothes. You don't need to slog on a treadmill or the jogging track. Just laugh toward a fitter and healthier you. According to Dr. William Fry, a professor of psychology and a pioneer researcher on laughter at Stanford University, ten minutes of hearty laughter is equal to thirty minutes on the rowing machine. This is with respect to cardiopulmonary endurance. Laughter yoga is ideal for busy professionals who have very little time to exercise. Twenty minutes of laughter yoga can give you results similar to that of one hour in the gym.

Aerobic Exercise

Laughter yoga exercises are devised to facilitate longer exhalation and deep breathing through the diaphragm. This helps to flush the lungs of stale air and increase the net supply of oxygen to the body and brain.

Increases Blood Circulation

Research studies have shown that laughter dilates blood vessels and improves pumping of the heart, thereby increasing blood circulation.[1] It is like internal jogging that massages and promotes circulation to the digestive and lymphatic systems. It flushes the body and organs of waste products, leaving us ready to perform our best.

Impact of Laughter Yoga on Belly Muscles: A German Study

A TV film in Germany showed one group of people doing laughter exercises and another group doing calisthenics. The objective was to do a comparative study on the impact of laughter yoga on the belly muscles. The study was conducted by Dr. Heiko Wagener, a professor at the University of Münster. And guess what? The laughter group showed greater mobilization of the low-lying muscles than the group doing calisthenic exercises. The participants of the laughter group belonged to the laughter club of Neuss (near Dusseldorf) and were led by Veronica and Gisela Dombrowsky.

This research was targeted to see the impact of laughter exercises on the abdominal muscles. Those who suffer from backaches have weak abdominal muscles, which lead to a protruded belly. This puts additional pressure on the spine, leading to herniation of disks and spasms in the back muscles. Those suffering from chronic backaches are advised to do abdominal toning exercises. The German study showed that laughter exercises activate abdominal wall muscles better than crunches.[2]

18

Laughter Yoga for Healing: Therapeutic Effects

"I have not seen anybody dying of laughter.
I know millions who are dying because
they are not laughing."

People who practice laughter yoga regularly report a significant improvement in health. Their blood pressure and blood sugar levels stay under control and the number of pills they take is reduced. Those suffering from arthritic pain do not feel the need to take painkillers while others say that they sleep better without sedatives.

At my clinic, I started making patients laugh after handing them a prescription and encouraged them to keep doing laughter exercises at home with their family. Surprisingly, I noticed that they healed faster and wanted to learn more exercises when they visited next. This made me believe that laughter had therapeutic effects.

As a doctor, I know that 50 percent of all illnesses are due to an organic cause, for instance the hardening of blood vessels in hypertension and the deficiency of insulin in diabetes. The other 50 percent are psychosomatic reactions like "what will happen to me," "how long will it last," "how much will I suffer." This is where laughter yoga helps. It creates a healing environment in the body by reducing stress levels and boosting mood.

According to psychoneuroimmunology, our mind plays an important role in manifestation and healing of a disease that has both mental and physical components. Laughter being a positive energy takes care of the mental component instantly and creates a positive environment for the healing process to begin. The therapeutic and healing effects of laughter can be attributed to a strong immune system and increased oxygen levels in the cells.

Laughter Boosts the Immune System

A weak immune system is the major cause of almost all sickness. In fact, we end up spending a lot of money on prescription drugs while overlooking the natural coping mechanisms of the body.

A weak immune system is also responsible for the development of cancer. Laughter quickly increases immunoglobulin levels that help fight infection and increases the number of NK cells in the blood. According to Dr. Lee Berk, laughing makes the body stronger as T cells, NK cells and antibodies show increased activity.[1] Laughter should be combined with other forms of treatment to provide cancer patients with an improved quality of life and the best possible chance of survival.

Disease-fighting proteins trigger an increase in IFN, a blood chemical that transmits messages and stimulates the immune system. An increase in immunoglobulin A (IgA) aids defense against the entry of infectious organisms through the respiratory tract. In general, laughter builds resistance against infections by increasing the concentration of circulating antibodies and white blood cells in the bloodstream.

Oxygen for Healing

Oxygen is one of the primary catalysts for all metabolic reactions in the human body. Ongoing scientific studies show that a lack of oxygen is a major cause of most diseases. Laughter yoga flushes the lungs and oxygenates the blood and major organs, leaving one feeling energetic and free from diseases. Research has also shown that cancer cells are destroyed in the presence of oxygen. In fact, many parasites and bacteria don't survive well in the presence of oxygen, which is why an increase in the oxygen levels with laughter exercises is a great way to combat diseases.

Dr. Otto Warburg spoke about the role of oxygen in maintaining good health. According to him, deep-breathing techniques increase the flow of oxygen to the cells and are the most important factors in living a disease-free and energetic life. When cells get enough oxygen, cancer will not and cannot occur. Incidentally, Dr. Warburg is the only person to have won the Nobel Prize for medicine twice and to be nominated a third time.

Heart Disease and Hypertension

Modern day stressors and lifestyle changes have increased the incidence of heart diseases. Even as doctors and patients try to minimize the risk factors, scientific studies have proved that laughter is the simplest answer to a healthy heart. Hearty laughter is one of the fastest ways to accelerate heart rate and enjoy the benefits of an excellent cardiovascular workout and heart massage. Dr. Michael Miller, a leading heart researcher at the University of Maryland, discovered that laughter expands the blood vessels, promoting circulation and reducing blood pressure.

Scientific studies have also proved that just a few days of laughter exercises and deep breathing lowers blood pressure, thus reducing the risk of a heart attack.[2] It improves circulation and increases the supply of oxygen. According to research conducted in Bengaluru, India, a ten-minute laughter session can help reduce blood pressure by 10–20 millimeters.[3] Laughter may not be a cure, but it does help to reduce the frequency of medication and even stop it. Too much cholesterol in the blood can lead to the hardening and narrowing of arteries (atherosclerosis). A daily dose of laughter opens them up and allows the blood to flow freely to all parts of the body, thus preventing a cardiac failure.

Linda Le Vier, United States: It was in 2004 that I went from showing no symptoms of a heart disease to a transplant. I was diagnosed with blocked arteries and a bypass surgery was scheduled. I had seven stents put in and was in the ICU for nine and a half weeks with one complication following another. My son was told that I may spend the rest of my life going from a bed to a chair and back, but I am relieved that he did not tell me.

After a year of slow recovery, I knew I needed to do more than walking and eating correctly. I needed a medicine with no side effects for my spirit. I heard something about laughter groups and went to join one. After just one session, I knew I had found what I was looking for. It was then that laughter yoga entered my life, which made me come out with a lighter spirit and feeling of self-confidence. My sense of joy led to less notice of pain, regular exercising and an influx of new friends who had a positive outlook and often laughed at themselves and funny situations.

While my heart continued to weaken, my spirit grew stronger. I had terrible days with fluid buildup. On the day that I meekly asked my doctor if I would be eligible for a "handicapped" parking placard, he gently told me that I would benefit from a heart transplant. "What? You must think I'm really sick. That hadn't occurred to me." I had many complications, but I underwent a heart transplant in 2007 on April Fool's Day. It fits my personality perfectly ... Ha ha! My doctors said I did so well because of my "gratitude attitude." I would say that came from my experience with laughter yoga.

Laughter Yoga and Diabetes

Diabetes is emerging as a major health hazard worldwide. Japanese scientist Kazuo Murakami's experiment to ascertain the effect of laughter on blood sugar levels has affirmed that laughter has a lowering impact on it. Murakami identified twenty-three genes that can be activated with laughter. In addition, it also reduces the levels of cortisol, which is responsible for an increase in sugar levels, thereby lowering blood sugar and helping diabetics.[4] It also stabilizes the immune system, which, if weakened, can affect the production of insulin.

The following is the story of Vishwamohan from Vijaywada who fought his illness of over thirty years with laughter yoga exercises.

It is common to celebrate one's birthday but that was not the case with Vishwamohan. He celebrates his birthday on the day he joined the laughter club as he feels he got a new lease on life and was reborn after joining it.

Constantly troubled by illnesses, he had almost given up on life. From chronic diabetes, high blood pressure and cardiac problems to diabetic neuropathy, he had suffered immense pain and anxiety in the fifty-three years of his life. After a bypass surgery in 1999, he had to endure other health complications as well. Disillusioned by constant medication and rising stress levels, he decided to adopt an alternative method that would help him feel better. On January 14, 2002, he joined the local laughter club. Gradually, his life underwent a remarkable change. His health improved considerably as his ECG, blood pressure and blood sugar levels stabilized. He had never felt healthier. He firmly believes that laughter yoga nurtured him back to health.

Bronchitis and Asthma

Laughter has a positive impact on allergies, with many practitioners reporting improvement of some symptoms of asthma and chronic bronchitis. I remember a gentleman who was severely asthmatic and used to travel five to ten miles every day to participate in a laughter session. Since he started practicing laughter yoga, he told me that he had hardly used his inhaler.

The usual prescription for asthma and bronchitis is chest physiotherapy to remove mucous (phlegm) from the respiratory passage. Blowing forcefully into an instrument or balloons are among the common exercises asthmatics are asked to do. Laughter yoga does the same job more easily and at no cost. It increases the antibody levels in the mucous membranes of the respiratory passage, thereby reducing the frequency of chest infections. It also tones up the mucous-clearing system of the bronchial tubes. Frequent belly laughter empties your lungs of more air than what you take in, resulting in a cleansing effect similar to that of deep breathing. This can be especially beneficial for patients who suffer from emphysema and other respiratory ailments.

Cancer and Other Chronic Illnesses

Those suffering from life-threatening diseases not only go through physical pain but also face immense psychological trauma. Not just the patient but even the family, friends and caregivers need relief from the stress. A positive mental attitude greatly influences the course of the disease. We have had many members suffering from cancer, immune disorders, multiple sclerosis and other chronic diseases, who reported relief from their symptoms after practicing laughter yoga.

In the past, inspired by the research on laughter, many cancer patients tried to use humor in order to laugh away their tumor. But it is not easy to laugh in a situation like that. This is where laughter yoga has an advantage. Since it is a physical method, it is ideal for cancer groups that can practice laughter as a form of exercise with no need for humorous interventions. It may not cure the disease, but it definitely helps to enhance one's ability to cope with it and improve the chances of survival.

RosBen-Moshe: When I was diagnosed with bowel cancer at forty-one, I was devastated. But being a laughter therapist I knew that laughter would be an integral part of my healing and recovery process. Believe me, it was not easy to laugh, but laughter yoga taught me that there was always a ray of hope.

I thought laughter would come naturally to me, but the first session I attended after my diagnosis seemed to be forced. I felt trapped and helpless. I could hardly muster the courage to conduct a laughter session when in a few days I was scheduled for major surgery—a full bowel resection with a temporary ileostomy. All I wanted was to hide and cry.

But life changed on my forty-second birthday. I decided to laugh away my fear and anxiety. I outlined the social, emotional and physical benefits of laughter and even managed to lead participants in a session that comprised laughter exercises, deep breathing and clapping. I noted how in no time my laughter became real, as did theirs. I realized that the more we choose to smile and laugh, the more we actually rewire the brain to a constant state of calm, joy and awareness.

After the session, I asked the participants to share how they felt and was delighted to hear that, like me, they felt happier, lighter and less anxious and stressed. It was for the first time since the diagnosis that I felt an excitement for life, for living. I felt more prepared for the surgery.

A few days later, when I went to the hospital, I promised to take charge of my healing. Even though the circumstances were less than perfect, I believed that laughter and a positive mental attitude would help me. Even during recovery, I focused on the positive energy and kept laughing because optimal healing takes place when there is less stress on the body and mind. Laughter yoga does just that as it changes your perspective and promotes complete wellness.

On most days, even if it was the last thing I felt like doing, I practiced my daily laughter. I knew doing so would change my biochemistry. With full attention on my smile, I would take a deep breath and then exhale until it was as if every cell, every tissue, every muscle, every fiber of my being was smiling back at me. It was such a beautiful thing to do, to embody a smile and the magical feelings it brings: love, inner peace and pure joy.

It also helped reframe some of the more painful moments, infusing them with a little joy, which I knew would help change the way my mind remembered particular events. I even changed how I referred to my bowel reversal, choosing to call it a bowel reconnection as instinctively this felt so much more positive. Basically, I spent time focusing on everything positive and joyful.

My journey with cancer reaffirmed the principles that I had only preached until then. I actually put them into practice and reaped the benefits of love, joy and happiness. Healing through laughter set me on the path to everlasting positivity, changed my perception toward life and taught me how to accept and deal with adversity.

Laughter Yoga and Depression

Depression is the leading cause of disability worldwide and a major contributor to the overall global burden of diseases. More women are affected by depression than men. It is a combination of symptoms that interfere with the ability to work, study, sleep and eat. A disabling condition, it can affect a person many times during their life. You must have noticed that depressed people seldom laugh. However, people who laugh are seldom depressed.

Laughter yoga has helped thousands of people all over the world to overcome severe depression as it uses laughter as a physical exercise rather than using cognitive humor. This means that anyone can laugh, regardless of their state of mind and cognitive ability. It is not unusual for people who have suffered long-term depression to recover through laughter, even after years of antidepressants.

Laughter yoga creates a positive state of mind and fosters a hopeful attitude with increased optimism. This makes the world seem like a wonderful place full of fun and interesting people, with a great potential for achievement and happiness. In this state, one is less likely to succumb to feelings of depression and helplessness.

Laughter works as a mild antidepressant as it releases endorphins and serotonin, giving the body pain-relieving effects and the mind a feeling of well-being. It also boosts optimism, self-confidence and feelings of self-worth.

Depression-linked stress switches off body systems not required for a fight or flight response. These include the immune, digestive and sexual systems. Thus chronic stress or depression causes one to lose interest in activities that bring pleasure, including sex and food. The weakened immune system leaves one prone to illness and disease. Laughter yoga has the opposite effect on the body. It boosts the immune, digestive and sexual systems, thus restoring the pleasures of good food and sex and enabling the body to fight diseases.

Depression is often associated with physical pain, feelings of despair, loss of appetite, immobility, insomnia and cardiovascular problems. Practicing laughter yoga regularly helps to resolve most of these symptoms.

Dianne Theil McNinch: In January 1997, my thoughts about committing suicide became frequent. In April 1997, I was diagnosed with clinical depression. Over time, my condition deteriorated and I spent over $400 on medication each month.

I first heard about laughter yoga on the American TV show *Dancing with the Stars*. It seemed delightful. On April 11, 2007, I happened to see a laughter yoga session on *The Oprah Winfrey Show*. Before the show ended, I had signed up for the May Sierra Madre training and tried to find a local laughter group. The next day, I met Jeffrey, a laughter yoga teacher who guided me through my initial session. Just two months after my first laughter experience, my use of medicines had come down by 80 percent. In fact, I'm completely off medication now and end up saving a lot. I sleep better and people tell me that I look great, that too at the age of sixty-four. My life has undergone a remarkable change.

Anxiety and Panic Attacks

Mental and emotional stress triggers the body's arousal mechanism by stimulating the sympathetic system and producing physiological and biochemical changes that lead to anxiety and even panic attacks. It is apparent that one's state of mind directly affects breathing. When in a stressful state, the breathing pattern alters drastically. It becomes faster, shallower and irregular. Sometimes people even hold their breath under stress, which leads to an accumulation of carbon dioxide in the blood.

Laughter yoga provides an excellent cardiac workout and triggers a breathing pattern that provides significant respiratory benefits. It lowers the amount of residual air in the lungs and replaces it with oxygen-rich air. This reduces the level of carbon dioxide in the lungs, thereby reducing the risk of pulmonary infections. By shifting the breathing pattern from shallow to deep diaphragmatic breathing, it stimulates the parasympathetic nervous system, which is the cooling branch of the autonomic nervous system and the opposite of the sympathetic stress arousal system. This scientific phenomenon, coupled with the ancient yogic wisdom of breathing, makes this concept a unique exercise regime to relieve stress and anxiety.

Here is the incredible story of a woman who suffered from severe anxiety and panic attacks since eight years of age. Right from childhood she was plagued with intensely negative emotions that made her life miserable. Depressed and dejected for years, she had almost given up on life when she discovered the world of laughter yoga. Her life changed for the better and the attacks became less frequent.

Christina Watson, Canada: Believe me when I say that I was taken to a shrink at the age of eight. I was in a special education class in grade five and was diagnosed with learning disabilities and visual perception problems. I cried a lot and was always scared. I constantly complained of stomachaches and constipation and feared the reactions of other children. Even my brother called me a crybaby.

Little things were enough to set off a panic attack. In fact, after I left home for college the attacks became more frequent. I took the Early Childhood Education program, wanting to work with young children, but I had trouble being a leader. I ended up on medication as the panic attacks worsened. Though I had supportive parents, I could not help but feel depressed and fearful all the time.

The turning point came when I met Dr. Kataria. Laughter yoga helped me relax my mind and reduced the frequency of the panic attacks. Now, I'm at peace with myself. I can think clearly and have developed a positive viewpoint. It has helped me both physically and mentally.

I started laughter yoga in April 2006, and since then I have been doing all my exercises faithfully every morning in front of a mirror. Laughter yoga is the reason behind my happiness. I feel I can handle the stress of daily life without getting agitated. I used to wake up scared, but laughter yoga helped me get rid of my fears. My eyes look brighter and I feel less pain when I laugh and chant "ho ho" and "ha ha ha."

My mom, too, has noticed the remarkable changes. She finds me to be in a happy mood as I talk more about the positive things in life instead of dwelling on the negatives. I have also started singing in the church choir, which was unthinkable five years ago. Laughter yoga has improved my communication skills and boosted my confidence. In fact, my mother now calls me a social butterfly!

Laughter yoga also helped me deal with my father's death. The attacks came back when he died, and I went into depression. The exercises taught me how to cope with the tragedy.

Laughter yoga is keeping me well overall. I believe that if I stop practicing laughter yoga, I will again slip into a state of distress. It is now my mission to continue with this powerful coping tool to keep well forever.

Natural Painkiller

Pain is triggered by the nervous system. It can be caused by an injury, sickness and disease, or can be brought on by psychological reasons that, if not treated, can be extremely detrimental to one's mental well-being. Physical pain management is comparatively easier than managing psychological hurt, which can lead to stress, anxiety and depression. People harboring mental hurt, resentment and guilt are hardly able to laugh and express their emotions.

Laughter yoga is a universal remedy to aid the release of emotions and to reduce pain. It is unique as it approaches laughter as a physical exercise rather than using cognitive humor. It is not unusual for people who have suffered chronic pain to recover through laughter.

The moment we sense pain, our bodies become tense and we experience muscle contraction. The more our bodies tighten, the more intense is the pain. Laughter yoga releases endorphins, natural opiates that are more potent than equivalent amounts of morphine. These help in reducing the intensity of pain in those suffering from arthritis, spondylitis and muscular spasms. Many women have reported a reduced frequency of migraines.

Laughter is an effective pain medicine that costs little and has no side effects. Twenty minutes of belly laughter can reduce pain for almost two hours. It also increases pain tolerance. Many cases of people having gone through physical trauma and recovering without the use of painkillers have been documented—they just laughed it off!

> **Lucinda, Canada:** I used laughter exercises to relieve a nagging toothache. During an uncomfortable drilling episode, I decided to do some laughter exercises to ease the pain. Just five minutes of this helped me go through four minutes of totally pain-free drilling. The pain returned after a few minutes, but by then the procedure was almost finished. Besides alleviating pain, my laughter lightened the mood at the clinic.
>
> I also do laughter exercises in the elevator. Believe me, it takes the edge off.

Laughter Yoga and Arthritis

Laughter offers respite from arthritic pain and provides both physical and mental relief. Both arthritis and spondylitis are debilitating disorders with inflammation of the joints. Documented research has proved that laughter is a great workout to increase one's threshold for pain.

The combination of natural painkillers and laughter exercises makes laughter yoga a powerful tool for physiotherapy. Many practitioners have reported reversal of frozen shoulder and other movement limitations due to strokes, arthritis and injuries. The release of beta endorphins because of laughter causes the adrenal glands to manufacture cortisol, which is a natural anti-inflammatory agent.

Laughter yoga sessions also include an element of stretching that prevents the stiffening of joints and improves mobility, thereby preventing spondylitis and arthritis. Usually, people find it difficult to adhere to any form of physical exercise, but laughter yoga provides the motivation to keep their exercise routine regular.

19

Laughter Yoga for
Personal Development

"Laughter is a tranquilizer with no side effects."

—Arnold H. Glasow

Personal Benefits

Besides being the best stress buster, laughter yoga has also proved to be very effective as a personal development tool. It enhances mental skills and abilities that help a person improve his/her performance in every sphere of life. If you ask people practicing laughter yoga around the world about the benefits they received, the first thing they would say is that just fifteen minutes of laughter keeps them cheerful throughout the day. This sense of well-being comes from the release of endorphins, which improve one's mood instantaneously. It is a proven fact that if your mood is good, you will do your best in every sphere of life.

Laughter yoga increases the ability to laugh at the smallest of things. This happens because laughter exercises done in a group help develop a sense of humor and childlike playfulness, which enhances the capability to laugh.

How It Changed My Life

Over the past fifteen years, laughter yoga has undoubtedly helped add more laughter to my life. Earlier, I could hardly laugh at things that most people found funny. For instance, most of them would laugh while watching movies, but I would barely manage a smile. This was because I would question the reason behind the laughter. In fact, this habit becomes a hindrance when one wants to laugh. It is very difficult to laugh when the mind sets conditions on laughter. But with years of laughter yoga, I've learned to be playful and increased my capacity to laugh.

My focus is on not using my brain to laugh. When I was still practicing as a medical doctor, I always looked for logic behind what was funny and what was not. Only very funny jokes made me laugh. Laughter yoga helped me bring laughter out of my mind and into the body. I realized that physical playfulness led to a playful mental attitude and changed my perception of humor. Now, I can see the funnier side of most things. In fact, I can say that the secret behind my laughter is childlike playfulness. This inner child helped me laugh much more than what I used to when I was a doctor.

No longer inhibited, I developed the art of making others laugh too. Though still not good at telling jokes, I have learned to laugh. When I make mistakes, I start laughing at myself, which helps me connect with people. The truth is that nobody is perfect; people connect with me because they find me to be imperfect.

Before laughter yoga, whenever I laughed, my mouth would never open wide enough and I would keep my teeth clenched. I would feel the tightness around my jaw. Most of the laughter came from my throat. But when I started teaching people about belly laughter and how to use the abdominal muscles to laugh, I realized that if the mouth is opened wider, laughter comes straight from the belly. In doing so, you can feel the movement of the diaphragm and even learn to laugh louder.

Earlier, I would suppress my laughter because I was mindful of the people around me. With laughter yoga, I can say that both the quality and quantity of my laughter have improved, and I can now laugh more heartily and loudly. It has not only changed my life but also helped many others.

Here are some benefits of laughter yoga that can help improve your life:

Self-Confidence

Laughter yoga is a powerful way to enhance self-confidence as it helps to overcome inhibitions and awkwardness. Laughter and smiling not only help to communicate effectively but also create a safe environment for others to connect with you. This goes a long way in achieving success in business, personal and social life.

Laughing in a group in a public place helps to shed most inhibitions, and over a period of time you become more outgoing. Gradually, it builds self-confidence and helps to develop personality and leadership qualities. People who smile always do better, especially those in the field of sales and marketing as a smile is the most important tool for customer service. But perhaps this tool should be used warily as some people may be sensitive or fearful of loud laughter and it might be counterproductive.

Greg Govinda, Australia: Laughter yoga has the potential to change lives in just one session and is especially effective when practiced regularly. It brought many changes to my life and challenged me to face some hidden fears. It also helped me to let go years of grieving that I hadn't been able to shake off. This happens because laughter releases our unconscious attachment to things that hamper our health and well-being. It provides an environment where one can feel free and open up to the wonder of being in a joyful space with others. In due course, I experienced a strong self-confidence and told myself that I was okay "just the way I am." I found a great sense of inner peace. Though I still face the usual challenges, I find myself more willing and able to relax and "look at" what it is within me that is feeling challenged. Laughter yoga is a powerful tool that allows me to appreciate what I have.

Communication Skills

Laughter yoga significantly improves communication skills by limiting self-consciousness and hang-ups. Although I had few inhibitions because I had done a lot of theater, I was always anxious about my performance on stage. I felt nervous while making speeches and was afraid of making mistakes, but laughter yoga taught me how to communicate effectively. Today, if I make a mistake, I just start laughing, which makes the whole process easy for me as well as my audience.

Stress and negative emotions hamper communication skills and the motivation to communicate. Laughter yoga is the perfect exercise routine to counter this effect. As it induces unconditional laughter, it enables people to express freely. It generates positive feelings and eliminates negative thoughts. In fact, it is hard to remain in conflict with someone when you are laughing.

Power struggles cause us to focus on ourselves and ignore others. Laughter interrupts this cycle and allows people to be more open with each other. When we laugh with others, criticism and sarcasm seem to evaporate. We are not judgmental and are able to let people be themselves. It also makes us generous to a level where we feel better giving than receiving. In effect, it promotes goodwill and cooperation between generations, between those with opposing viewpoints, and even between nations.

Another important communication skill that one can acquire through laughter yoga is the art of maintaining the right amount of eye contact. If it's too little, it hints at lack of self-confidence, while too much eye contact can be intimidating. Though it is difficult to specify how long you should look into the eyes of another person, constant practice of laughter exercises can help you get it right.

P. T. Hinduja, Mumbai: I want to share my journey from being a company secretary to a laughter champion. I lived in the same building as Dr. Kataria in Mumbai. I was an introvert who hardly laughed. I used to deal with legal matters and barely had a sense of humor, but today I am a "laughter champion." This amazing transformation took place in 1995 when I joined Dr. Kataria's laughter club. I was hesitant initially, but when I saw so many people laughing together, I too joined them. I started enjoying my laughter and got better with every passing day.

In 1997, it was by sheer chance that I participated in a laughter competition. I had no choice as one participant was absent. To my surprise, I was adjudged the "best laughing man." My self-confidence got a boost, and I repeated the feat at the next laughter championship held in Goa during the first All-India Laughter Convention. When the people there asked me my secret, I told them that I did not laugh only as an exercise but that I really enjoyed it. Seeing my continuous winning spree, Dr. Kataria made me a judge.

Laughter yoga taught me to laugh more than I ever did. My sense of humor improved significantly. My stress levels have come down, and I'm full of energy throughout the day. Besides this, I have become much more generous. Earlier, I would get irritated at small things, but now I don't lose my cool easily. Laughter yoga has helped me express myself freely and stay positive. My level of satisfaction has gone up, and I don't react negatively to other people's behavior. Laughter yoga helped me the most when I was going through a tough phase of life. My wife was sick and bedridden for nearly two years. At that time, laughter helped me cope with the situation.

It is never too late to join a laughter club. One can learn to laugh at any age. I joined one in my seventies and am an active member even in my nineties.

Maintains Emotional Balance

It is comparatively easy to manage physical or mental stress compared to emotional stress that arises due to problems at home, work, relationships and strained situations. Faced with such circumstances, people find it hard to express their feelings. Laughter yoga helps emotions to flow and releases pent-up feelings. It defuses emotions like fear, anger and resentment, thus preventing conflicts, easing tension and helping one understand the other person better. Not only does it release negative emotions, it also cultivates unconditional love, generosity, openness, compassion and the willingness to help others.

Emotional Intelligence Through Laughter

All of us have some basic needs, desires and aspirations. There are certain things that give us happiness. Then there are things that get in the way of our goals. Emotions are what we use to express what we want and refuse what we don't want. We express emotions through thoughts that take the form of words, which finally motivate us to take action.

Emotional intelligence is the ability to process emotions the right way. It is the capacity to recognize not just our own feelings but also those of others. It helps to motivate us and manage our emotions in the best possible manner without hurting ourselves or others. Normally, we do two things: we either express or suppress emotions. Expression of emotions may lead to conflict with others, while suppression can harm an individual. The right form of expression has a positive impact and leads to an appropriate action whereas repressed emotions get logged in our subconscious mind and can lead to negative physical repercussions.

Most people carry the baggage of unexpressed emotions that can wreak havoc in our bodies. Laughter yoga allows one to release these emotions from the subconscious mind. For instance, many people may reflect sadness on their face, not because of something that has happened in the recent past but because of something that may have happened a few decades ago or perhaps in their childhood. They may have undergone some negative experiences that they may not remember. Unconditional laughter helps to release this unknown baggage and attain emotional balance.

Many people act on an impulse, which can lead to regret. Emotional and impulsive decisions can help a person achieve heights or land them in serious trouble.

The role of emotional intelligence is to develop a person's ability to think and rationalize the consequences before acting on an impulse. People who have well-developed emotional skills are usually more productive as they have mastered the art of controlling their feelings while taking important decisions in life, whereas people who do not have this ability are more prone to wrong decisions and poor choices.

Laughter yoga and deep-breathing exercises change the sympathetic response of fight or flight to the parasympathetic mode, which can easily be activated through deep diaphragmatic breathing and belly laughter.

Liz Morfea, United States: I was always a melancholic child. After being sexually abused by a stranger, followed by my dad committing suicide when I was six, I retreated into my mind, which was the only place I felt I had control. This often resulted in obsessive-compulsive behavior, dissociation from reality, anxiety and depression.

Following the birth of my son in 2005, I experienced severe post-partum depression and post-traumatic stress. It was during this time that laughter yoga found me. I went to a laughter club and thought: "This is fun, I feel good, but I don't really get it." I did not realize then that there was really nothing to "get," nothing to comprehend. It was only the will to surrender to the simplicity of it all.

Laughter yoga gave me the confidence I never knew before. It has connected me to greater joy and possibilities. I not only laugh more, I am also able to express all emotions more freely: hurt, disappointment, anger, sadness and happiness. It remains my therapy. I truly believe in laughter yoga as an empowering tool to fight depression, mental illness and trauma.

Laughter yoga enabled me to feel peace and compassion and has given me the clarity to know my own boundaries. My proudest laughter yoga achievement so far is sharing it with a man currently serving a long sentence in a high-security prison. He has, in turn, taught other inmates this technique and formed three weekly laughter clubs in prison, which have had a profound effect on the relationships among the prisoners and also reduced violence.

20

Laughing Through Challenging Times

"All your pain will become 'champagne'
if you learn to laugh for no reason."

Laughter yoga goes beyond just laughter. It not only fosters a feeling of physical well-being but also enhances the spirit and touches the emotional core of those who practice it.

In times of difficulty, it is not easy to remain calm. By imbibing the inner spirit of laughter yoga and its characteristics, one can learn to handle situations without losing composure. It creates a new experience each time that enables one to handle similar situations in the future.

People are often surprised at the powerful changes that laughter yoga brings to their lives. The ever-present ego and the "I" mellow down to a loving, caring and giving state of mind. It alters a selfish character into an altruistic one. It cultivates a positive mental attitude and an understanding based on unconditional love, forgiveness, generosity and compassion. It allows virtues of patience and tolerance to emerge.

Laughter helps people to develop a state of emotional fluidity where worries and goals become less important. The inner spirit of laughter ensures that people around us are also happy. It is important that as we seek our happiness, we remain mindful of bringing happiness to others too.

Laughter has taught me the true meaning of spirituality: "if you can raise your spirits by yourself and raise someone else's spirits too, you are spiritual."

The following narratives reaffirm how laughter yoga helps people to maintain a positive attitude in the face of challenges.

- **Anita Aggrawal, India:** I joined a laughter club in April 2015 when I was suffering from hip bone and lung cancer and was confined to a wheelchair. After joining this club, I saw a drastic change in myself. My health improved, I put on weight, I could walk with the walker and even drag my wheelchair to the club. Not just this, I could also do laughter yoga while standing for almost half an hour. Over time, I have been able to do my daily chores and become independent. I feel as if the cancer has been cured. My husband, who has seen the change in my health, continues to encourage me to go to the laughter club. Everybody is so affectionate; I have no words to express my feelings for all the members. Thanks to laughter yoga, I now look forward to life. It has worked wonders for me!

- **Junsuke Ando, Japan:** I would probably have died many years ago had it not been for laughter yoga. But here I am, in my seventies, very much alive and kicking. Laughter yoga saved me from three cerebral strokes, a heart attack, bankruptcy and a divorce. It gave me a new lease on life and an inner strength to cope with all the challenges I faced. It brought back my lost laughter and hope and filled me with positivity and joy.

I want to share my story with as many people as possible so that those who are critically ill and suffering may be rescued from their pain and sorrow by laughing. I am convinced that laughter makes us healthy, both physically and mentally.

I suffered my first stroke during a lecture in 2002. I could not speak and my right side was paralyzed. Thanks to the rehabilitation program, I got my speech back. But it was the physical immobility that made me self-centered and irritable. My wife was unable to cope with my selfish behavior and left me, which threw me into depression. This lasted almost three years even though I underwent psychiatric treatment. In 2004, I was officially acknowledged as a physically handicapped person by the Tokyo municipal government. It was as if my life had stopped and I had nothing to look forward to.

Five years later, in 2007, I suffered a second stroke. The right half of my body was paralyzed again though I did not lose my speech. The paralysis, however, remained and the after-effects of the stroke were obvious in my clumsy movements.

Two years later, in 2009, I came across laughter yoga. I was at a restaurant when a rather elderly lady approached me. She must have sensed that I was ill and began talking to me about laughter yoga, explaining how it combines deep breathing and laughter to bring about a substantial change in the body. She even demonstrated a couple of laughter exercises, but I was rather indifferent. In spite of understanding my disinterest, she gave me her card, which proved to be the turning point in my life.

When I understood that laughing indeed was good for health, I decided to call the number and go to the Tokyo Olympic Center to meet Mary Tadokoro, who managed a laughter yoga club. In the first encounter, I explained my physical condition. I knew that I could not do any exercise that would require difficult movements. Mary told me to just sit on a chair and watch everyone.

When I came home after the session, my blood pressure had come down, which I found very strange as I had not actually participated in laughter yoga. Mary then told me that even if you do not laugh, just being in the same place as laughing people leads the brain to think that you are laughing. I decided right there to try laughter yoga out. It was not easy to force laughter, but in a very short period of time the sense of embarrassment faded away and I found myself laughing with the group. Two months later, I did a leader training course and met Dr. Madan Kataria, who said that in order to get all the benefits of laughter one must make it a habit. From the very next day, my daily laughing began. I have not missed a day since. It's been almost eight years.

Gradually, my health improved. But in 2012, I suffered a third stroke. The doctor told my brother that I may not survive. Again, the right half of my body was paralyzed and I had trouble speaking. I accepted that I may be nearing my end.

Although the doctors said that I would have to be hospitalized for six months, I was able to leave in three months. This was because of the cheerful atmosphere created by my laughter yoga friends who visited me daily. Once it became possible to stand up, I went to several laughter yoga clubs in a wheelchair so that I could be surrounded by the energizing laughter. This helped in my recovery.

But my travails were not over. In 2014, I suffered an angina attack and had to be hospitalized once again. The doctors said I needed immediate surgery as my arteries were clogged. Though everyone felt it would be better to get the operation done quickly, my laughter friend Yuriko had a different opinion. She said, "You are still alive although your blood vessels are all worn out. If you get a surgery, it may just kill you on the spot." I opted out of the operation and decided to focus on laughter yoga. And then a miracle happened. The doctor told my friends that a very strange thing was happening. Right next to my clogged blood vessels, new ones were growing. This was unbelievable! Laughter yoga, my friends and my determination to live had combined into a great force.

In appreciation of laughter yoga, I started a club so that more people could benefit from this movement. For me, laughter yoga is the medicine that works on life. I feel great now; I can do almost anything. As a septuagenarian "laughter phoenix" who wants to repay the universe for the great miracle that laughter yoga bestowed on me, I know I will live many, many more years—laughing, thanking and loving. I know that I am not the only one to be convinced of this truth. I know you will be too. Ha ha!

- **Laura Gentry, United States:** A few days after my mother's hip replacement surgery, she reported some unusual symptoms to my dad, who took her to the emergency room. They discovered that she had a life-threatening aortic aneurysm. It was decided that she would be transported by a med-flight to a hospital nearby for an emergency heart surgery.

As we anxiously waited for the procedure to end, I called the organizer of an event for which I had to do a laughter yoga program the next day. I had made a commitment to open the conference for the postmasters of Iowa with rollicking laughter. But in that moment of crisis, laughter was the last thing on my mind. The organizer couldn't find a replacement speaker but offered to let me off the hook so I could stay at the hospital with my family.

Amazingly, my mom made it through the surgery. Since the rest of the family was there and she wouldn't regain conscious that day, my sister urged me to go ahead and speak at the conference.

What an incredible day it was! Being able to bring joy and laughter to a mob of postmasters was just the lift I needed in that difficult time. They were so grateful that my husband and I had come. Many of them didn't even know that my mom was in the ICU.

After the conference, I returned to the hospital and spent some quality time with my mom. She was aware and appreciative of our presence. Two days later—after we had left for the night—she lost consciousness and could not be revived. My mother died on the Mother's Day weekend.

My life changed. The sadness was overwhelming. I didn't how I would overcome this loss.

The day after her funeral, however, I was at the laughter club. People thought it odd that I could laugh, but I said, "How can I not laugh? Laughter is healing and life-giving. I need to practice laughter yoga all the more in the depths of my grief."

As the months went on, I added more laughter to my routine. I began spending half an hour each morning doing the breathing and laughing exercises. It revitalized me and gave me the strength to grieve. In addition, the laughter yoga community supported me. I could feel the tangible power of their love as they continued to pray for me. I credit laughter yoga with giving me the ability to walk through this dark valley to the light and happiness on the other side.

Lalla Laura Ribaldone, Italy: My life collapsed in 2013 after my husband fell ill and later divorced me. I was accused of leaving him because of his sickness. Many people hurt me, which led me to consider suicide. I needed a caretaker because I am deaf and was living all by myself.

Having no parents or relatives to rely on, I cried a lot. I even contemplated taking up a job but being deaf kept me from doing so. I felt I was a burden and no longer wanted to live. Then, in May 2016, I came across laughter yoga, which led me to join a laughter club. Initially, I was not very convinced but I continued to attend sessions. Gradually, I started feeling better and felt some small changes. I realized that I was not crying any more; on the contrary, I found myself laughing.

Laughter yoga helped me rediscover lost emotions and I learned to love myself. In short, it uplifted me and taught me to review my problems positively. Though I still face some discomfort in the evening when I come home and find no one to welcome me, I am beginning to deal with these situations better.

I have to thank all my laughter teachers who have helped me achieve this state of happiness. Today, I am a much better person who has many friends. I feel at peace with myself and am happy to confess that laughter yoga encouraged me to face my fears, mostly related to my deafness. I am more confident and ready to take on all of life's challenges with a smile.

Part V

APPLICATIONS OF LAUGHTER YOGA

21

Laughter Yoga at the Workplace

"Take your work seriously, but take yourself lightly."

—Bob Nelson

People today face tremendous stress and risk burnouts at the workplace. Even highly talented and skilled people cannot perform well if they are emotionally unstable. Though there are many other ways to reduce stress, laughter yoga addresses most of the workplace-related issues in a cost-effective and time-efficient manner. It is a single exercise routine which reduces physical, mental and emotional stress.

By introducing laughter yoga sessions for their staff, companies have reported increased efficiency, better communication, increase in sales and productivity, increased creativity and better teamwork, decrease in illness and absenteeism and a reduction in employee turnover.

Three Types of Work Stress

Physical stress results from working beyond one's capacity. Working continuously without sufficient rest makes one tired and exhausted.

Mental stress stems largely from heavy workloads with tight deadlines, from fear of losing one's job or pushing too hard to fulfill basic needs. Competing with others or yourself to improve performance also leads to mental stress.

Emotional stress is deep-rooted and triggered by bad relationships at home or at the workplace. Emotional problems at home reflect at work and vice versa. Emotional stress is more difficult to cope with than physical and mental stress. One can deal with it at two levels:

- **Develop Skills to Express Emotions Freely:** Laughter yoga helps to develop emotional expression through physical playfulness and a playful mental attitude. While playing, you focus entirely on the process while the personality takes a back seat. One is creative, dynamic and full of fun. Most people spend a lot of time and energy holding on to their masks and personalities. Physical playfulness helps to shed all of these and enables free expression of emotions.

- **Increase One's Ability to Release Pent-up Emotions:** Suppressed emotions cause physical or mental pain and affect performance. Laughter yoga provides a simple, painless and effective release mechanism to help rid the subconscious mind of pent-up emotions. This helps to build performance and improves intelligence and communication skills.

Peak Performance

In this highly competitive world, everyone wants to stay ahead and be the best. We have to work regardless of our state of mind or mood. The good news is that you can quickly change your mood within minutes by doing laughter yoga exercises.

A positive state of mind is essential to determine your energy and enthusiasm levels. Your mood mainly depends on your emotional balance and the ability to handle positive and negative emotions. If your emotional balance is negative, you will generate more negative emotions, which will lead to stress, depression and low energy levels. On the other hand, positive emotions release endorphins and put a person in a good mood.

Did you know that positive emotions can be created by the use of movements because of the two-way link between the body and mind? By doing laughter and breathing exercises, one can kick-start the good hormones that elevate the mood instantly. This changes your perception of the world, thereby improving performance in every field. Another way that laughter yoga helps to optimize performance is by increasing the levels of oxygen in the body and brain.

Team Building

"People who laugh together, work together," said John Cleese, a renowned British comedian, during his visit to Mumbai. Laughter is a great connector as it breaks all hierarchies. It is a powerful tool that helps develop a positive mental attitude, hope and optimism and increases communication skills, all of which are prerequisites for team building.

A laughter yoga group session allows people to share and care about one another. It provides a sense of emotional security, which resists stress and promotes excellence in all areas of life. Laughter yoga teaches one to understand others and balance emotions. It diffuses stress and generates peace and harmony in the mind, which leads to improved thinking and creativity. Team goals become clear and accepted by everyone, even as they learn to complement and balance each other instead of building conflicts. It promotes a strong connection between those who laugh together, resulting in family-like bonds. It connects people without being judgmental and enhances leadership qualities, thereby creating an atmosphere of openness.

Mirror neurons in the brain cause us to experience the emotions of those we communicate with. Laughing with people helps us experience their laughter. Each time we establish eye contact with people who are laughing, the mirror neurons add their laughter experience to our own, which creates a feeling of togetherness—a major component for successful team building.

In a pressurized work environment, people succumb to hierarchy, status, competitiveness and a feeling of insecurity that hampers constructive potential. It leads to feelings of low self-esteem and fear of performance. Laughter yoga provides group interaction, which helps to diminish these feelings and boost confidence levels.

Laughter Yoga: A Quick Recharge Mechanism

It is not possible to work continuously without taking breaks. Working hard constantly calls for quick recharges to help revive energy levels. According to the ultradian rhythm of the body, one cannot work with the same output for more than ninety minutes. Performance starts to decline after this and goes on decreasing for almost twenty minutes. The attention span and concentration levels fall and efficiency gets affected. People then look for distractions such as smoking, going for a walk, etc. This pattern can get restrictive during training schedules, meetings, seminars and conferences.

Seriousness at the Workplace

Like laughter, seriousness is contagious. If the head of a company is serious, the team members are likely to be that way too. Seriousness rubs off on colleagues and clients. However, it is not conducive to efficiency and creativity. One may achieve targets but meaningful growth gets retarded. This explains the phrase "take your work seriously, but take yourself lightly." If you don't have any idea about how to overcome your seriousness, simply start laughing and being playful and see your seriousness turn into joyfulness. Laughter yoga encourages one to indulge in playful activities until our body develops the intelligence to create a new behavior of playfulness that helps to dispel seriousness.

Eye Contact and Smile: Tools of Communication

In the business world, developing the art of smiling and maintaining eye contact is the most effective way of communicating. Smiling people do better business, especially in sales and marketing. Laughter yoga has proved to be extremely beneficial in this respect as the whole concept is based on making each other laugh just by eye contact.

Innovation and Creativity

The childlike playfulness cultivated by laughter yoga stimulates activity in the right side of the brain, which is the seat of creativity. This helps generate new ideas and insights about workplace issues and problems. As one needs to introduce innovative ideas constantly in order to stay ahead, laughter yoga allows people to be more creative and original.

Playfulness in business settings may not be possible in a spontaneous way as it needs to be structured and organized. People need to make a commitment and get involved in playful activities to develop their creative skills and improve the work ambience. Laughter yoga helps to develop playfulness in a subtle way. Moreover, when practiced in a group, it provides a safe environment to do so.

With repeated sessions, playfulness gets wired into the body and mind and becomes a part of one's psychological makeup. This soon starts reflecting in day-to-day activities, even during office hours. It provides a safe environment to introduce schemes, make strategies, set up discussions and debates, develop common visions and replace old assumptions with fresh ideas.

Value of Laughter Yoga for Professionals

People working in the business world are exceedingly busy and have no time to exercise. Also, because most exercises are a lot of hard work and tend to get monotonous, people abandon the programs altogether. However, laughter yoga is a powerful exercise routine with a difference. There are no postures or skills to learn, no special yoga clothes or equipment required, and since it is done in a group, it is easy to learn. Anyone can do it and become an expert.

It has been proved that ten minutes of hearty laughter is equal to thirty minutes on the rowing machine. This is not in term of muscular movements but cardiopulmonary endurance. The purpose of all aerobic exercises is to stimulate heart rate, increase blood circulation, supply oxygen and remove waste products, thereby improving mental and physical health. And there's nothing better than laughter yoga, which is a complete wellness exercise routine.

Positive Work Environment

Job dissatisfaction and a hostile work environment compel people to change jobs frequently, which affects productivity and profitability. Laughter yoga creates positive energy and improves communication between people. Our research in Bengaluru in 2006 concluded that laughter yoga triggered an increase in positive emotions among the participants. This helped to create a more constructive work environment and ensured loyalty and commitment.

- **Effect of Laughter Yoga on Stress and Emotions (Bengaluru Study):** In December 2006, S-VYASA, Bengaluru, conducted a scientific research involving 200 IT professionals to study the effects of laughter yoga on stress. Seven laughter yoga sessions were conducted for half the group over an eighteen-day period with physiological, immunological and psychological tests performed on each person before and after the laughter yoga sessions. The study was undertaken by one of India's leading scientific research organizations.

The Result

- **Decrease in Blood Pressure:** The 6 percent reduction in systolic blood pressure is significant and suggests reduced sympathetic nervous system activity or reduced stress levels. The 4 percent reduction in diastolic blood pressure is also significant and suggests relaxation. There was no change observed in the control group. The significant reductions in blood pressure indicate that laughter yoga helps reduce stress and improves ongoing stress management.

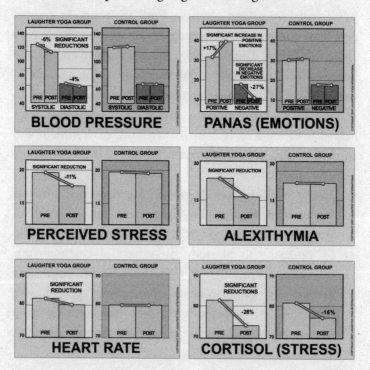

- **Reduced Cortisol:** There was a 28 percent reduction in cortisol levels in the laughter yoga group and a less significant change in the control group. Early morning cortisol levels were measured for both groups before starting and after completing the laughter interventions.

PANAS (Positive Affectivity and Negative Affectivity Scale)

This test assesses the emotional style a person uses to cope with events. Negative emotions such as fear, disappointment, distress, upset, sadness, guilt, nervousness, shame and misery decreased by 27 percent for the laughter yoga group.

There were no significant changes for the control group. This strongly indicates that laughter yoga reduces negative emotions, which results in improved communication skills, better workplace motivation and a more positive outlook.

Perceived Stress Scale (PSS)

The PSS measures an individual's perceived stress. Both groups were measured before and after the laughter interventions. There was an 11 percent reduction in perceived stress in the laughter yoga group as against a small change in the control group. This points toward significant stress release, which equips the laughter yoga group to handle stressful events better.

Alexithymia

Alexithymia is a serious condition in which people have difficulty identifying and expressing emotions. People with a high alexithymia scale tend to fight with others frequently, are cold and distant in their behavior, are socially inhibited, experience anxiety in the presence of others, show a lack of initiative and have difficulty coping with social challenges.

Alexithymia is the opposite of emotional intelligence. It reduces empathy, communication skills, creativity and innovation—all of which are skills that are identified as critical for success at the workplace. Our tests showed a significant 8 percent decrease in alexithymia within the laughter yoga group after seven sessions as against no change in the control group.

Impact of Laughter Yoga on Workplace Efficacy: U.S. Study

Another study conducted in the United States in 2007 looked at the effects of laughter yoga on personal efficacy at the workplace. It involved thirty-seven participants from a behavioral and mental health facility in the Midwest.[1]

Self-efficacy is the belief in one's ability to organize and take action to achieve a goal or manage a situation. This personal belief influences the choices people make, the effort they put into working toward a goal, how long they persist when confronted with obstacles and how they feel during the process of working toward goals. Self-efficacy beliefs affect performance at the workplace.

Personal efficacy testing was done for the participants the week before, the week after and sixty to ninety days after a series of daily laughter yoga sessions. Laughter yoga was practiced for fifteen minutes daily for two weeks.

The results showed significant improvements for the laughter yoga group in all areas. It is particularly interesting to note the long-lasting effects of the laughter interventions.

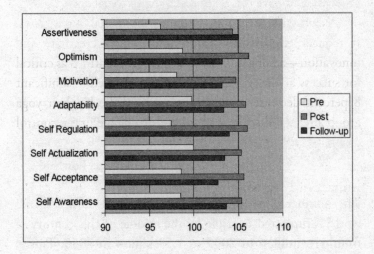

22

Laughter Yoga for Seniors

"You don't stop laughing because you grow old.
You grow old because you stop laughing."

—Michael Pritchard

The number of people above sixty-five years of age in the world is projected to triple by the middle of this century—from 516 million in 2009 to 1.53 billion in 2050. This is because of advances in medical science that have led to a rise in life expectancy and created a population of senior citizens who long for emotional comfort and solace.

As the joint family structure gives way to nuclear set-ups, the elderly, particularly in the West, find themselves alone in old-age homes where they hardly laugh and smile. Though they live with people their age and there is a community feeling, they yearn for a family. All they need is someone to talk to and friends to share their emotions with. What better than laughter to help them, which offers both—the much-needed sense of fellowship and a connection with people.

As we grow older, we laugh less. Dementia and Alzheimer's disease leave the elderly unable to understand jokes or find anything funny. This is because humor is a mental and cognitive phenomenon. Laughter yoga works for them as an exercise because of the multiple health benefits it offers.

Retirement Blues

When the laughter yoga movement began in India, most participants were the elderly. They can be divided into two categories: those who have just retired and are physically active and those living in old-age homes and assisted living centers. When people retire, they have all the time to relax, enjoy and do what they want. It feels great for a while, but soon they get bored and try to look out for some meaningful social activity that lets them spend time with other people. With advancing age, they develop health problems. Some resort to gambling, drinking and other addictions. Laughter yoga becomes a boon as it helps reduce stress, generates a positive attitude, boosts self-esteem and assists in overcoming the feeling of insecurity.

Lack of Bonding

The elderly are always in need of human contact. While most of them are surrounded by like-minded peers, they still miss a family. They crave for someone they can share their feelings with. Laughter yoga sessions have the power to reach beyond the healing of laughter. The effective network of caring-sharing relationships is the key to a happy and healthy life. Relationships with people become strong and the feeling of loneliness dissipates. Seniors enjoy the daily meetings as it generates a sense of belonging. Laughter yoga can give seniors the much-needed feeling of closeness and fraternity.

Decline of Cognitive Faculties

Faced with age-related issues, the elderly find their physical and mental faculties worsening. The degeneration of brain cells makes it difficult for them to understand and organize facts, let alone humor. Simple tasks become difficult, leading to rising frustration, which makes it harder for them to laugh. Under such conditions, laughter yoga helps the elderly reap the scientifically proven benefits of laughter to improve health and well-being. It provides an emotional bond and is one of the most powerful tools against depression.

Since it can often be difficult for the elderly to understand humor, laughing as an exercise is much easier for them to enjoy its benefits. Laughter yoga helps them live a life full of joy again. Being a physical process, it does not require any mental abilities, thus helping the elderly to understand humor without using cognitive faculties. A few hours of laughter every day improves memory, thinking ability and intellectual capacity.

Promotes Physical Health

Most seniors have ailments such as high blood pressure, diabetes, asthma and other age-related diseases. Laughter yoga helps to strengthen the immune system, increase oxygen supply to the cells and produce a positive mental state. Regular practitioners with chronic pain, migraines, headaches and asthma have found the attacks to become less frequent, and in some cases to disappear completely. Many with high blood pressure, severe spinal, neck or shoulder problems, and even diabetes, have found their life returning to normal without the need for medication.

Laughter Yoga Makes Exercise Programs Interesting: U.S. Study

Normally, seniors abandon their exercise programs due to lack of motivation. An interesting study conducted at Georgia State University under Dr. Jennifer Craft Morgan and laughter yoga teacher Celeste Greene showed that incorporating laughter into a physical activity program can improve the confidence levels of the elderly in their ability to exercise.

For six weeks, the participants attended two forty-five-minute physical activity sessions per week that included eight to ten laughter exercises lasting thirty to sixty seconds each. A laughter exercise was typically incorporated after every two to four flexibility exercises. The study found that 96.2 percent of the participants found laughter to be an enjoyable addition to the program. They reported that the program enhanced their motivation to participate in other exercises or activities and improved mental health and aerobic endurance. The findings were published in the journal *The Gerontologist* in November 2017.

Improves Circulation

Lack of mobility often leaves the elderly complaining of cold hands and feet. Laughter yoga exercises the lungs and circulatory system and pushes the heart rate up to a level comparable to any other aerobic exercise. Laughter yoga is an ideal workout for the elderly as they cannot walk and do much physical exercise because of weak muscles and arthritic problems.

Insomnia Among the Elderly

Many elderly people who had difficulty sleeping and needed tranquilizers and sleeping pills found laughter yoga exercises helpful in getting good quality sleep. It was once thought that high levels of cortisol led to insomnia, but a 2003 study suggested that the opposite was true. Chronic insomnia— which is often caused by chronic stress—produces higher levels of cortisol. The Kyungpook National University, Korea, conducted a study in September 2007 that involved 109 men and women over the age of sixty-five. It found that just four laughter therapy sessions in a month were associated with more restful sleep and reduced feelings of depression. Insomnia is so common that nearly one out of every two people complain of poor sleep. Not only does insomnia adversely affect productivity and emotions but also increases the risk of depression, hypertension, metabolic syndrome and heart diseases.

Supports Good Mental Health

Many seniors suffer from depression, frustration and anger. As they lose loved ones and health, it becomes increasingly difficult to maintain a positive mental attitude. Laughter yoga changes a person's biochemistry in a way that supports good mental health regardless of circumstances.

Laughter Yoga Prevents Strokes

Advancing age and hardening of the arteries, commonly known as atherosclerosis, impede the flow of blood and trigger angina, which can result in full blockage, heart attacks or strokes. Similar blockage of the arteries in the brain can cause cerebral strokes, leading to paralysis. Laughter yoga exercises help to reduce bad cholesterol, control blood pressure and prevent platelet aggregation, minimizing the chances of a heart attack and stroke.

Effect of Laughter Yoga on Stroke Patients: Research in South Africa

Dr. Gita Suraj-Narayan, a senior lecturer at the School of Social Work and Community Development, South Africa, and a laughter yoga teacher was inspired to carry out research exploring the biopsychosocial impact of laughter therapy on stroke patients. The study used laughter yoga with cognitive restructuring as an alternate form of therapy. It began in September 2008 and comprised 120 laughter therapy sessions that used various laughter techniques, pranayama and cognitive restructuring. The participants included stroke patients between the ages of forty and ninety years.

Significant Findings of the Study

- A reduction in post-stroke depression that was the result of direct damage to emotional centers in the brain. Compounded by frustration and difficulty in adapting to new limitations, it included anxiety, panic attacks, flat affect (failure to express emotions) and apathy, often characterized by lethargy, irritability, sleep disturbances, lowered self-esteem, withdrawal and a reduction in stroke-related pain.

- Enhanced mobility and the ability to move around without walking aids.

- Endorphins released as a result of laughter helped in reducing the intensity of pain.

- In some cases, laughter therapy helped patients recover from cognitive issues like perceptual disorders, speech problems and issues with attention and memory.

- Improved communication between the patient and the family.

23

Laughter Yoga for Schoolchildren

"Unless you turn and become like children,
you will never enter the kingdom of heaven."

—Matthew 18:3

Many people believe that when a child is born, he/she mirrors
the natural human state before the realities of the world modify
behavior and state of mind. If this were true, then humans
would always be naturally joyful and healthy. But this is not
the case. As we grow up, our ability to laugh and play decreases.

Earlier, children would spend their childhood playing
and developing emotional skills, which we call emotional
intelligence. This playful behavior resulted in laughter and
happiness.

Sadly, children today are faced with several pressures. They
are faced with many stressors and have forgotten how to laugh
and play. Physical activity is restricted, new strains are imposed,
adult behavior is demanded at an early age and group play
and child-to-child interaction has been replaced with electronic
games and remote communication devices. What is needed is
a system that is integrated into educational institutions, which
helps them cope with stress and find time for play and laughter.

With growing awareness about the benefits of laughter, many schools are incorporating laughter yoga into their curriculum. Several high school books have chapters on laughter yoga. For example, the Grade 10 CBSE English course book, the Japanese high school book *Pow Wow,* and the language course book at Cambridge University have a chapter on the origins and benefits of laughter yoga. What we need is incorporation of laughter yoga exercises in schools on a regular basis. It is the best way to bring more laughter into the lives of children and make them stronger, both mentally and physically.

Laughter yoga was formally introduced in schools in India in 1998 and since then has spread informally to schools in Mumbai, Bengaluru, Surat and other Indian cities. It was observed that students felt more energized, their attitude and communication improved, their willingness to learn and innovate increased, disciplinary problems were reduced and a gradual decrease in sickness and absenteeism was noted. There was a significant change in the atmosphere of the school and many teachers said that it had brought a meaningful change to their attitude and re-energized and re-motivated them.

Why Children Need to Laugh More Today

- **Academic Pressure**: Children, whose energy was traditionally expressed through movement, laughter and play, are being forced to sit still and concentrate for extended periods from an early age. Faced with a competitive academic environment, they are pressurized by parents and teachers to score well. High expectations, at times, lead the children to strive for unrealistic goals, which if unfulfilled can bring on serious stress and prove to be detrimental to their mental and physical health.

Studies show a huge increase in cases of attention deficit hyperactivity disorder (ADHD). Children with this disorder find it difficult to concentrate for even short periods. They act on impulse and often appear to have no sense of danger.

- **Technology Robs Them of Play**: Physical play is being replaced by mobile phones, video games, television and the Internet. High-tech communication devices have eroded the fun of laughing at simple things.
- **Lack of Emotional Bonding:** More and more broken families and the consequent lack of emotional bonding and long-term relationships with parents combine to cause a host of emotional problems. Working parents and a reduction in family size leaves children alone for long periods of time, devoid of the parents' presence. This leaves the children deprived of moral and emotional guidance.
- **Negative Attitude Toward Laughter in Schools:** Children are often programmed against laughter. Teachers ask children to stop laughing in the name of discipline and sometimes even punish them. In such a case, the children learn that laughing is not good, which is one of the reasons they lose their laughter as they grow up. Apart from schoolkids, there is also a large population

of teenagers faced with the demands of college life and pressure from parents to achieve goals that may be unrealistic. Not meeting these goals often leads to anxiety and in some cases even suicidal tendencies.

Benefits of Laughter Yoga for Schoolchildren

- **Developing Emotional Intelligence:** Modern studies show that children develop emotional intelligence through laughter and play. Those who don't play enough in their childhood grow up emotionally unstable and find it difficult to maintain relationships. In fact, emotional intelligence is now being recognized as the single major factor contributing to long-term success. It is play that helps to develop emotional and social skills and teaches one to cope with situations. However, children today stay glued to their mobile phones, televisions and computer screens. Laughter yoga encourages children to go out and play and express themselves fully. Childlike playful behavior is the key to developing emotional intelligence.
- **Improving Academic Performance**: Oxygen is food for the brain. Lack of oxygen affects brain functions such as concentration and leads to confusion and dizziness. Laughter exercises flush the lungs of stale residual air, which helps kids to concentrate better, increases learning ability and helps to enhance academic performance.
- **Boosting Immune System**: Regular laughter exercises reduce absenteeism due to cough, cold and chest infections by boosting the immune system.

- **Building Stamina:** Laughter yoga increases stamina, which is required in both schools and colleges, by increasing breathing capacity.
- **Developing Confidence**: By encouraging self-expression through laughter exercises, children can find their own voice. Their leadership skills and self-confidence grow as laughter yoga exercises remove inhibitions.
- **Enhancing Creativity**: As laughter yoga has play at its core, it triggers activity in the right side of the brain and enhances creativity.

Three Models of Laughter Yoga Program for Schools

- **Assembly Session:** Many schools in India and other countries have incorporated a five-minute laughter yoga session during the morning assembly. Since the number of students present for the assembly is big, the impact of laughter exercises is profound. It becomes evident in the energy levels of the children throughout the day.
- **Laughter Yoga in a Classroom:** Schoolteachers can also conduct laughter exercises for a few minutes either at the beginning or end of their classes. My team and I also tried doing laughter exercises just before the children went home and found that it made them happy and energetic. The parents also reported that they came back smiling.
- **Laughter Yoga Rooms**: We have set up laughter yoga classrooms at Vidya Prakash High School in Bengaluru where we conduct thirty-minute classes to teach students

the basics of laughter yoga, brain gym exercises—a series of coordinated movements of the hands touching different parts of the body—as well as how to combine singing, dancing and laughing. We also asked the students to teach these exercises to their parents and other family members.

Laughter Yoga with Teenagers

Teen stress is an important health issue. We know that the early teens are marked by rapid physical changes.

Teenagers laugh a lot with their peers but are not so open during their interactions with adults. They go into a shell and want to play it safe. They are afraid of feedback and are extremely awkward. On the threshold of adulthood, they are afraid of facing the challenges of growing up.

Major Teen Stressors

- **Puberty:** A child changes physically and emotionally with the onset of puberty. Even their attitude toward the parents undergoes a change. Often, children think their parents are annoying and old-fashioned. In return, parents may find the child to be cheeky and sullen. It is a time of conflict, but it is more alarming not to have any trouble at all. It might be indicative of the fact that the child is hiding his/her problems, which can affect the psyche. Extended hearty laughter induced by laughter yoga is extremely beneficial as it helps to release pent-up feelings.

- **Parental Inconsistency**: During this transitional phase, parents raise their expectations and can become inconsistent in their behavior. Sometimes they want their child to behave like a kid and sometimes like an adult. It is common to hear parents say "Don't do this, you are a kid" or "You can do this, you are big enough." These instructions send confusing signals to the child, leading him/her to become self-protective. Laughter helps to dissipate distrust and hostility arising out of continuous confrontations with parents. The release of endorphins kick-starts good feelings and changes the mood almost immediately.

- **Changing Relationships:** Puberty is a time when the child begins to feel liberated, but support from the parents remains paramount. Parents are not only a safety net but also the platform from which the child eventually experiences the world. Laughter helps to boost self-confidence and encourages a network of healthy relationships. It encourages team building and eliminates feelings of aggression, jealousy and antagonism.

- **School Demands:** As teenagers step into adulthood, they experience a changed environment. The new-found freedom brings with it pressures of performance, competitiveness and search for excellence. This leads to stress, which can even prove to be fatal. Laughter has the ability to reduce stress and provide a feeling of wellness.

- **New Responsibilities:** As teenagers become older, they take on new responsibilities. Hearty laughter helps to develop a sense of independence and self-reliance. It boosts self-esteem and helps them perform better in every sphere of life.

Laughter yoga is a very economical addition to any educational institution. Training costs are low and the major investment is time. Because laughter yoga is fun, it is normally welcomed and enjoyed by both the students and the staff. No known downsides or side effects have been reported. It is a physical exercise that works on the body and mind simultaneously. It stimulates willingness to learn and improves creativity and self-discipline. It provides tools to deal with stressful situations in new ways, besides offering an alternative to anger and aggression.

Laughter indeed is the best medicine for both young children and teenagers. In fact, in the educational context, laughter is used to prepare students for examinations and to encourage sports teams to perform well.

24

Laughter Yoga for People
with Special Needs

"He deserves Paradise who makes his companions laugh."

—The Koran

Living with disabilities can be hard to deal with. It can lead to severe mental trauma and stress and leave individuals prone to negative emotions that undermine rationality, giving rise to a confusing mind-set regarding one's own capabilities. Also, feelings of self-pity and self-worthlessness set in.

Laughter Yoga with Mentally and Physically Challenged People

Laughter yoga has the ability to elevate the mood and help a person cope with physical and mental disabilities, while providing relief from negative feelings. The group dynamics of laughter yoga lead to more openness and help people to accept reality, making it a great technique to maintain emotional balance.

Many people with physical disabilities are unable to move much without regular physiotherapy. Due to lowered mental functions, they often find it difficult to follow commands. Laughter sessions help them be more compliant with physiotherapy commands, leading to notable improvement in motor functions. Also, because the exercises revolve around laughter, all physical challenges are approached positively. Participants do the best they can and feel that they have succeeded because they are invited to laugh on their own terms. Such a situation is a win-win.

Benefits of Laughter Yoga for the Disabled

- **Relieves Pain:** Laughter triggers endorphins that provide immediate pain relief. What is worth noting is that people's relationship with pain shifts as they find that they can laugh at what was earlier a source of physical and emotional hurt.
- **Dissipates Anger:** Life is not fair, and neither are physical disabilities. "Why me" is a nagging question many people with disability ask themselves. Trying to live with a disability can be very frustrating as it forces one to be dependent on others. Choosing to laugh allows one to disconnect from the past and focus on the present.
- **Alleviates Sadness and Depression:** People with disabilities have to endure years of hardship and suffering. They often find it hard to express their emotions, which leads to depression. Laughter yoga helps to alleviate negativity.
- **Lowers Stress and Anxiety:** Any form of disability can be a cause of immense stress and anxiety. Frustration,

anger, aggression and irrational logic overcome the power of reasoning. Laughter has been shown to provide a substantial and immediate reduction in stress levels by lowering the levels of cortisol and epinephrine and enhancing the levels of health hormones and neuropeptides.

- **Helps to Express Emotions:** Physical incapacity can put people in a state of shock and trauma. There is not just physical pain but also denial, which can lead to feelings being blocked. Group dynamics in laughter yoga sessions lead to more openness and help people to share their grief. The exercises and the deep breathing relax the body and the mind.

Laughter Yoga with the Blind

Normally, we laugh in a group and stimulate each other through eye contact. But with the blind, we need to hold hands and verbally teach them the movements of different laughter exercises. As visually impaired people are talented in creative fields like music, weaving and other arts, combining laughter with music makes for a great arrangement. It leads to a joyful state of mind. We have introduced laughter yoga in many blind schools in India, Japan and Taiwan and the results have been positive.

Deaf Mute Children

In India, we have implemented laughter yoga programs in many deaf mute schools and got excellent results. Since the primary issue with these children is hearing, their speech too is impaired. One of the techniques we use with them is: follow the leader. We instruct them with the help of a sign language teacher who the children try to mimic.

Other common techniques include warm-up exercises to open up their voice—a kind of yodeling like "aaaaeeeeoooo"—accompanied by body movements, "ho ho" and "ha ha ha" actions and different laughter exercises. This helps the children to express themselves more clearly by altering the pitch and tone of their voices.

We were pleasantly surprised at the amount of laughter sounds they generated, which their staff in charge had never heard. The children remained happy throughout the day, and we found a significant improvement in their speech after regular laughter exercises. There are three schools in India in Nasik, Udaipur and Mumbai where laughter yoga has been implemented on a regular basis.

Laughter Yoga with Prisoners

Some years ago, actor John Cleese had come to Mumbai to shoot a BBC documentary titled *The Human Face*. The laughter clubs of India were a part of that series. During his visit, I took him to Arthur Road prison for a laughter session with the prisoners, which was a humbling experience. An hour before the session, I went to the overcrowded jail to build a rapport with the inmates. As I explained the concept, about seventy to eighty prisoners opted to join the laughter session. I was not too sure about whether they would laugh because they looked sad, angry and depressed. Some of them had mask-like faces. After initial hesitation, they opened up and laughed as if all their anger had transformed into laughter. At the end of the session, everybody seemed happy and asked when they would laugh like this again.

I spoke to many prisoners after the session and realized that they harbored a lot of repressed anger and depression that needed to be eliminated in order to prevent them from committing more crimes after being released. Laughter yoga is the ideal method to resolve these long-standing negative emotions in criminals. Introducing laughter in prisons worldwide will not just help the prisoners but also the jail staff, warden and others who constantly live under pressure and stress.

Laughter Yoga with Police Personnel

Faced with an ever-increasing crime rate, the police are under constant stress even though yoga and meditation camps are organized regularly for them. I was once invited to conduct a seminar at the Police Academy in Nashik and Vadodara. In the beginning, it was very difficult to make the policemen laugh in front of their seniors, but once they started laughing the session worked out well. Another factor that was a hindrance was that looking serious and tough is a part of their job. Laughing without a reason was hard initially, but after the session I saw them visibly relaxed.

Laughter Yoga with Multiple Sclerosis

Multiple sclerosis attacks the brain and affects the ability of the nerve cells in the brain and the spinal cord to communicate.

Though there is no known cure for this, laughter brings about positive changes and chemical reactions in the brain that can benefit patients. Studies have repeatedly found that laughter has both physiological as well as psychological benefits. It not only makes them feel better, it also helps the body heal.

25

World Laughter Day: Mission World Peace Through Laughter

"If people around you are not happy, they will not allow
you to be happy. Much of our happiness depends on
our ability to spread happiness around us."

The vision and mission of the laughter yoga movement is to bring good health, happiness and world peace by making people laugh. The World Laughter Day, which I thought of in 1998, is customarily celebrated on the first Sunday of every May. On this day, laughter club members and their friends and families get together in public places to laugh and send out positive vibrations and unconditional love, kindness, compassion, tolerance, understanding and forgiveness.

Today, we need to laugh more than ever. Surrounded by a sea of negativity with violence, terrorism, natural disasters, global warming, bad economy and other factors, it has become almost a challenge to remain happy and healthy. Laughter is a positive and powerful emotion that has all the ingredients required for individuals to change themselves and the world.

How Can We Bring World Peace Through Laughter?

The wars and conflicts that we see are a reflection of the wars going on in the minds of people all over the world. Unconditional laughter has the power to change our inner chemistry and make us feel good inside, thereby changing the way we see the world. This is where laughter yoga offers a solution. It is the easiest, safest and the most cost-effective solution for physical, mental, social and spiritual well-being. It contributes powerfully to maintaining health and happiness of individuals.

Laughter is a universal language that has the potential to unite humanity. Laughter yoga is a powerful tool to connect people from different cultures and countries. Through this movement, we create a community of like-minded people who believe in unconditional love, laughter and joy. If people from around the world come together to share a common vision of love, compassion, appreciation and forgiveness, it is possible to create an international community.

Collective Aura

Laughter is a powerful emotion that creates a positive aura around individuals. When a group of individuals laugh together, it creates a community aura. Electromagnetic waves from a group of individuals laughing every day form a protective layer around that area. The day that even 1 percent of the world's population starts practicing laughter yoga will be the day when global consciousness changes.

Tiffany Floyd, United States: I was overweight and my reproductive system was essentially dormant. I was diagnosed with amenorrhoea at twenty-seven after having only two menstrual cycles in four years. My sleep was erratic and my energy levels remained low. I would constantly ask myself questions like: Am I in menopause already? What if I can't have babies? Do I have cancer? Do I have diabetes? Is this my life now?

After doing laughter yoga sessions during my training in India, I started menstruating, which was a major healing breakthrough. It was like a release from the past.

Even as I kept up my laughter practice, medical tests revealed that the cysts in my ovaries were dramatically shrinking in size. My joints were moving freely for the first time in months and I was more flexible than I had ever been. I lost 35 pounds without dieting! Laughter yoga helped me find myself. I feel happier and lighter.

Laughter Yoga Being Practised Around the World

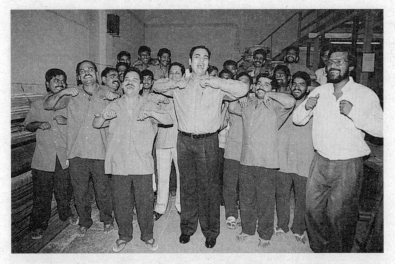

Factory workers during a laughter yoga session in Mumbai.

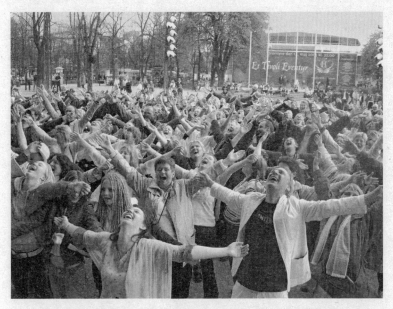

A laughter yoga session in progress at Copenhagen, Denmark.

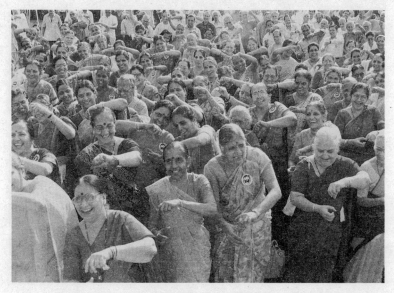

Members of a laughter club in Dombivli near Mumbai.

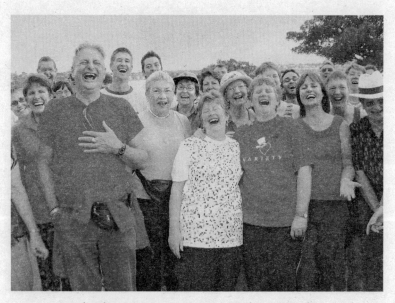

A laughter session in progress in Sydney, Australia.

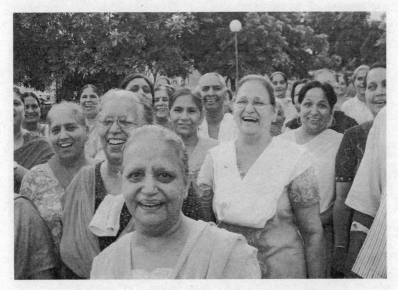

Members of a laughter club in Chandigarh, India.

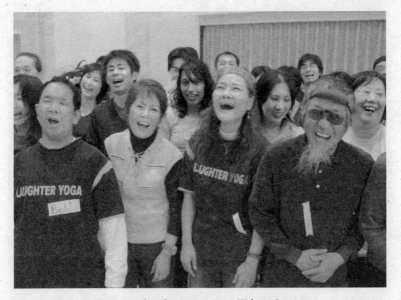

During a laughter session in Tokyo, Japan.

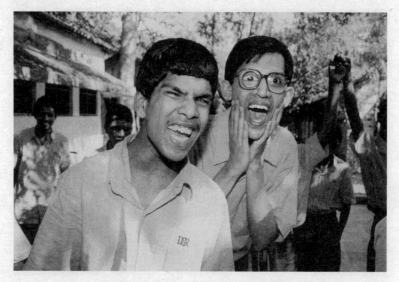

A laughter session in progress at the National
Association for the Blind, Mumbai.

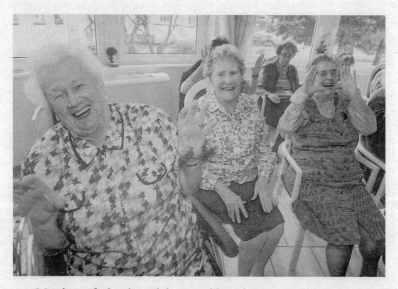

Members of a laughter club at an old-age home in Soultz, France.

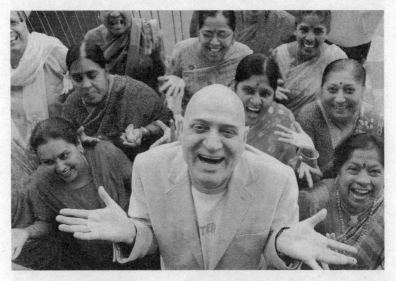

At a laughter yoga club in Bengaluru, India.

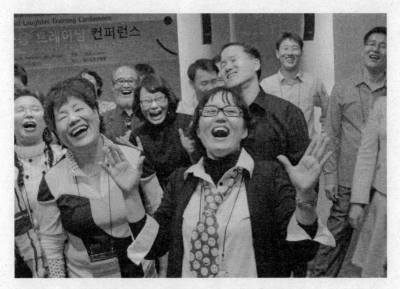

Professionals participate in a laughter yoga
session in Seoul, South Korea.

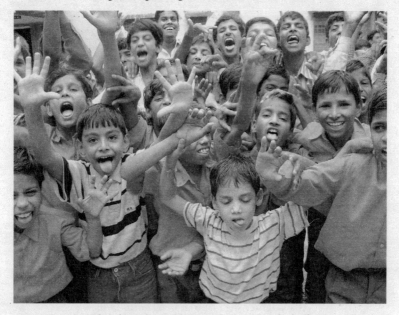

A laughter yoga session in progress with deaf-
mute children in Udaipur, India.

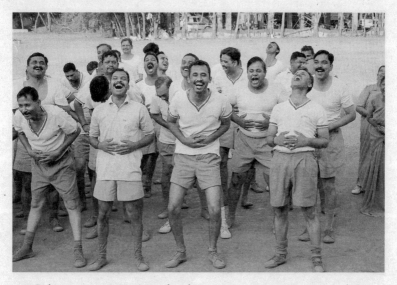

Policemen participate in a laughter yoga session in Gujarat, India.

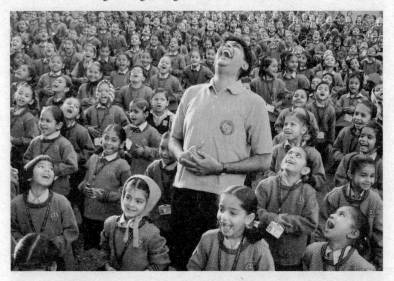

Schoolchildren during a laughter yoga session in Surat, India.

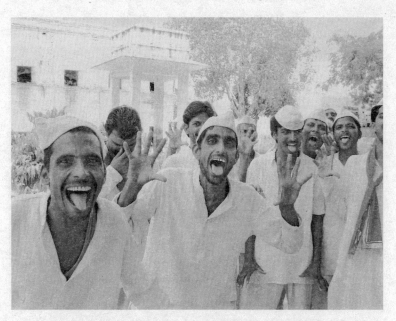

A laughter session in progress at the Udaipur Central Jail, India.

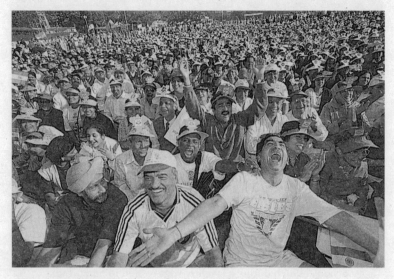

World Laughter Day being celebrated at Shivaji Park, Mumbai, in 1999.

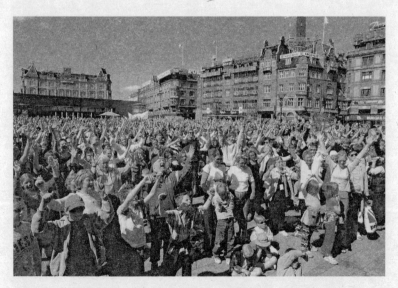

World Laughter Day being celebrated at Town Hall Square,
Copenhagen, in 2001.

Afterword

How often do you wish for more laughter in your life? How often, when you see others laughing heartily, do you wish you had a reason to laugh as well? One of the reasons the frequency of daily laughter is declining is because laughter has been left to chance. We cannot be passive spectators waiting for something to make us laugh. We need to make a commitment and be actively involved in bringing more laughter and joy in our lives. Otherwise, it may be too late.

Everyone has a choice. If you choose to be sad, nobody can stop you; if you choose to laugh, no one can stop that either. Life itself has no real meaning; personal choices dictate its meaning and outcome. The decision to glide through trying times with a smile or laugh is entirely your choice. So why not decide to laugh?

The core teachings of laughter yoga are: know laughter, do laughter and be laughter. Try it and see the difference for yourself.

Know Laughter

In order to bring more laughter into your life, be aware of its benefits. Ongoing scientific studies, plus the success of the laughter yoga movement, have proved that laughter has a powerful and profound effect on the body and mind. Not only does it help to prevent illnesses but it can also contribute toward healing chronic diseases: both physical and mental. Understanding the benefits of laughter will motivate you to get involved in laughter yoga exercises.

Do Laughter

Knowledge alone is not enough; you have to practice laughter to experience the benefits. After you decide to bring more laughter into your life, you will face several obstacles. As it happens in life, there will be the naysayers, those whose mission is to discourage and dissuade. They will question your motive and remind you that life is serious and not a laughing matter. My advice is: believe in laughter, believe in its healing value and believe that it can change your life. Then go ahead and do it.

Be Laughter

This is the ultimate stage of laughter, which teaches you how to actually live it. It is when you can take laughter with you wherever you go. Laughter should reflect from your ever-smiling face. It should become evident from your words, behavior and attitude. You should not only laugh during good times, but also keep your spirits high through challenging times. This can happen only by consistently practicing laughter yoga and making it an integral part of your life. It happened to me and I am sure it will happen to you. All the best with your laughter life!

Appendix

More Laughter Exercises

Swinging Laughter (Arm Swinging): Stand holding hands in a wide circle. Upon instructions from the leader, move toward the center by mimicking the prolonged vowel sound of "aay, aay, aayyyy." After a bout of laughter, move back to the original positions. The second time, move forward while saying, "eeee, eeee, eeee." Similarly, the third time, you can say "ooo, ooo, ooo."

Appreciation Laughter: This is a value-based laughter where the leader reminds the participants of how important it is to appreciate others. Join the tip of the index finger with the tip of the thumb, making a small circle. Move your hand forward and backward, looking at all the other members and laughing gently, as if appreciating them. After this, chant "ho ho" and "ha ha ha" and clap.

You can also use the thumbs-up position to look at the others and laugh.

Forgiveness/Apology Laughter:

a) Indian Way: Cross your arms and hold your ear lobes with the index finger and thumb. Bend at the knee, bow down and laugh.

b) Western Way: Spread your arms out as if saying sorry and laugh.

Laugh at Yourself: Point one finger toward your heart and laugh. Move around and look at other people as if you are laughing at yourself. This is the best ego busting exercise.

Laughter Cream: Pretend to squeeze a tube of cream on to your hands, or scoop it out of a jar. Then apply it on yourself and the others and laugh.

Wi-Fi Laughter: Place your index fingers on your head in a way that they resemble antennae trying to catch Wi-Fi signal. Walk around laughing.

No Money Laughter: This precedes the jackpot laughter. Pull your pockets out and laugh holding your palms out as if you have no money.

Jackpot Laughter: Imagine you have won a lottery. Start jumping and laughing as if you have become rich.

Waxing Laughter: Pretend to apply wax on your forearms thrice. The fourth time, pull it off as if removing hair from your arms. You can do the same on your legs and laugh.

Laughter Center: Point a finger to your head as if trying to find the brain's "laughter center." Alternately, you can also point to other body parts and laugh.

Crowded Elevator Laughter: Pretend you are in an overcrowded elevator. Stand shoulder-to-shoulder with the others and make different laughter sounds.

Laughing at Aches and Pains: Point to any part of your body that hurts (it could be your knee, back, stomach, shoulder or neck) and laugh your pain away.

Household Chores Laughter: Keep laughing as you pretend to do household chores like washing the dishes, using the vacuum cleaner, cleaning windows and folding clothes.

Sports and Games Laughter: Imitate movement of different sports and games while laughing. You can try weightlifting, shot put, discus, javelin throw, archery, boxing, karate, swimming, volleyball and baseball.

Head on Belly Laughter: Lie down on your back, with the bodies of other members at right angles to yours (place your head on someone's belly and have someone else's head on your belly) and laugh.

Ants in Your Pants Laughter: Run around laughing as if your pants were full with ants.

Balloon Laughter: Take some balloons. Kick and bounce them on your knees like a Hacky Sack. Every time someone makes contact with a balloon, they must laugh. This is a real workout and can keep you laughing for a while.

Hot Sand Laughter: Tiptoe as if you are walking on hot sand and react to the heat by laughing, running and carrying on.

Ice Cube Laughter: Pretend you are putting ice cubes down each other's backs. Be playful and laugh.

Laughter Ball: Play catch in pairs or as a group. Throw an invisible laughter ball to one another. Whoever holds the ball laughs. You can also dribble the ball and laugh each time it hits the floor. Sometimes it works well to use a real ball. A soft one is best.

Laughter Pill: Take imaginary laughter pills and laugh, and then try each other's pills. You can try the "over the counter" variety for a snicker or "prescription strength" for a big laugh.

Library Laughter: Pretend you have a case of giggles and are in a library. Try to keep your laughter down.

Hot Potato Laughter: Sit in a circle and pass an invisible hot potato around as fast as you can, laughing when it is in your possession.

Mental Floss Laughter: Pretend to hold a flossing thread. Move your hands to either side of your head as if flossing your brain and laugh.

Notes

Chapter 2: What Is Laughter Yoga and Why Do We Need It?

1. "Depression," World Health Organization, http://www.who.int/mediacentre/factsheets/fs369/en/.

Chapter 3: The Essential Link Between Yoga and Laughter

1. Richard A. Brand, "Biographical Sketch: Otto Heinrich Warburg, PhD, MD," National Center for Biotechnology Information, https://www.ncbi.nlm.nih.gov/pmc/articles/PMC2947689/.

Chapter 5: The Concept and Philosophy of Laughter Yoga

1. James D. Laird and Katherine Lacasse, 2014, "Bodily Influences on Emotional Feelings: Accumulating Evidence and Extensions of William James's

Theory of Emotion," *Sage Journals*, https://doi.org /10.1177/1754073913494899, published online on December 17, 2013.

Chapter 6: Voluntary vs. Real Laughter

1. Robert Provine, 1996, *Laughter: A Scientific Investigation. American Scientist*, "Contagious Laughter: Laughter Is a Sufficient Stimulus for Laughs and Smiles," 1992, *Bulletin of the Psychonomic Society*, Vol. 30, Issue 1, pp. 1–4.

2. Giacomo Rizzolatti and Laila Craighero, "The Mirror-Neuron System," *Annual Review of Neuroscience*, Vol. 27, pp. 169–92, https://doi.org/10.1146/annurev.neuro .27.070203.144230, first published online on March 5, 2004.

3. E. Foley, R. Matheis, and C. E. Schaefer, 2002, "Effects of Forced Laughter on Mood," NCBI (U.S. National Library of Medicine National Institutes of Health).

4. Paul Ekman, 1990, "Voluntary Facial Action Generates Emotions Specific Autonomic," *Psychophysiology*, Vol. 27, Issue 4.

Chapter 10: Cultivating the Habit of Smiling

1. Daniel Wiswede, Thomas F. Münte, Ulrike M. Krämer, and Jascha Rüsseler, 2009, "Embodied Emotion Modulates Neural Signature of Performance Monitoring," https://doi.org/10.1371/journal.pone.0005754.

Chapter 15: Four Strategies to Bring More Laughter into Your Life

1. Joe Verghese, Richard B. Lipton, Mindy J. Katz, Charles B. Hall, Carol A. Derby, Gail Kuslansky, Anne F. Ambrose, Martin Sliwinski, and Herman Buschke, 2003, "Leisure Activities and the Risk of Dementia in the Elderly," *New England Journal of Medicine*.

Chapter 17: Laughter Yoga for Wellness

1. Dr. Michael Miller, 2011, "Laughter Has Positive Impact on Vascular Function," European Society of Cardiology.
2. Heiko Wagner, Ulrich Rehmes, Daniel Kohle, and Christian Puta, 2013, "Laughing: A Demanding Exercise for Trunk Muscles," *Journal of Motor Behavior*, http://dx.doi.org/10.1080/00222895.2013.844091.

Chapter 18: Laughter Yoga for Healing: Therapeutic Effects

1. Lee S. Berk, David L. Felten, Stanley A. Tan, Barry B. Bittman, and James Westengard, 2001, "Modulation of Neuroimmune Parameters During the Eustress of Humor-Associated Mirthful Laughter," *Alternative Therapies in Health and Medicine*.
2. Dr. Michael Miller, 2005, "Laughter Helps Blood Vessels Function Better," *Science Daily*.

3. M. S. Chaya, M. Kataria, and R. Nagendra, 2008, "The Effects of Hearty Extended Unconditional Laughter," American Society of Hypertension.

4. T. Hayashi and K. Murakami, 2003, "The Effects of Laughter on Post-Prandial Glucose Levels and Gene Expression in Type-2 Diabetic Patients," American Diabetes Association.

Chapter 21: Laughter Yoga at the Workplace

1. H. Beckman, N. Regier, and J. Young, 2007, "Effects of Workplace Laughter Groups on Personal Efficacy Beliefs," *Journal of Primary Prevention*.